BASIC HEALTH PUBLICATIONS USER'S GUIDE

TO HEART- HEALTHY SUPPLEMENTS

Learn About the Most Important Nutrients and Supplements for a Healthy Heart.

MICHAEL JANSON, M.D.
JACK CHALLEM Series Editor

The information contained in this book is based upon the research and personal and professional experiences of the author. It is not intended as a substitute for consulting with your physician or other healthcare provider. Any attempt to diagnose and treat an illness should be done under the direction of a healthcare professional.

The publisher does not advocate the use of any particular healthcare protocol but believes the information in this book should be available to the public. The publisher and author are not responsible for any adverse effects or consequences resulting from the use of the suggestions, preparations, or procedures discussed in this book. Should the reader have any questions concerning the appropriateness of any procedures or preparations mentioned, the author and the publisher strongly suggest consulting a professional healthcare advisor.

Series Editor: Jack Challem
Editor: Susan Andrews
Typesetter: Gary A. Rosenberg
Series Cover Designer: Mike Stromberg

Basic Health Publications User's Guides are published by Basic Health Publications, Inc.
www.basichealthpub.com

CONTENTS

INTRODUCTION

Heart disease (specifically arteriosclerotic heart disease, or ASHD) is the number-one killer in the United States and other developed countries. Quite often, sudden cardiac death from a heart attack is the first indicator that a problem exists, so it is important to take preventive measures before the first sign of a problem. Most of the time, heart disease is the result of poor lifestyle choices, such as smoking, excessive alcohol intake, poor diet, lack of exercise, and high stress levels. This is actually good news, because it means that it is something that you can influence by making the right choices.

When I was in my first year of college in 1962, I was asked to undergo a routine evaluation by a cardiologist because I had had a heart murmur all of my life. I had always been told that the murmur was "routine" or "functional," and not significant for heart function. As it turned out, my prior evaluations were incorrect, and my heart murmur was indicative of a leaky valve that I had probably had since birth. Needless to say, this was quite a shock to both my parents and me.

At that time, the cardiac surgeon told my parents that he wanted to do surgery to replace the leaky valve that was causing the murmur. Although I had absolutely no symptoms, he said to them that if I did not have this done, I would likely have heart failure in ten to twenty years, when the heart muscle could no longer keep up with the increased burden created by the leak. He also urged me to give up any exercise,

even though I was a very active teenager and partic-
ipated in many sports.

We did not take his advice. However, it did stimu-
late my interest in heart health, and medicine as a
career, and in later years my interest in alternatives to
conventional treatments (and how to take better care
of my heart). This personal interest has kept me
aware of the most important developments in the
management of heart disease for myself and my
patients. While it is true that genetic makeup contributes to the development of heart disease, this is
far less important than lifestyle choices over which
you have a large measure of control.

Even if you have a family history of heart disease
(or almost any other chronic, degenerative disease),
do not feel that you are inevitably going to have the
same problem. Extensive research shows that diet,
exercise, stress, and many other influences play a
role in maintaining a healthy heart or contributing to
its decline, depending on the choices that we make.
In addition, the scientific literature is quite clear that
many dietary supplements are valuable as either
complements to conventional care, or in many cases
as substitutes for medications and even surgery.

CHAPTER 1

NORMAL HEART FUNCTION

In order to appreciate the value of dietary supplements for the heart, it is helpful to understand the basic structure and function of the heart. After all, your heart pumps all day every day of your life, and it cannot "take a breather" at any time, so it is well worth a few minutes to review how it does its work. However, it is not essential to understand how the heart works in order to benefit from the dietary supplements and other lifestyle changes presented later in the book. If you want to skip to the section on the valuable supplements for heart disease, you can always come back to the basics later.

Heart Anatomy and Function

The heart is a muscle much like any other muscle in your body, with some microscopic differences. This muscle, or myocardium, is a specialized sac with four interconnecting chambers. The right atrium and left atrium chambers receive blood that is coming back from the body and the lungs, respectively. Blood that has given up some of its oxygen to the tissues and picked up some waste products of metabolism comes into the right atrium from the vena cava, the largest vein in the body. From the lungs, blood that has picked up oxygen comes back to the left atrium through the pulmonary vein.

The left atrium then pumps some blood through a valve called the mitral valve into the left ventricle (although most of the blood actually passes through without the need for the pumping action, the atrial contraction does contribute significantly to the blood in the ventricle). The left ventricle then pumps oxygenated blood out through the aortic valve into the aorta, the largest artery, and then to the rest of the tissues and organs of the body (other than the lungs). While the left ventricle contracts (an event called "systole"—pronounced "*sis*-tuh-lee"), blood is prevented from going back into the left atrium by the mitral valve. When this blood passes through the kidneys and liver, waste products and toxins are removed.

Blood that comes into the right atrium passes into the right ventricle through the tricuspid valve, and during systole the right ventricle contracts sending blood to the lungs through the pulmonary valve and the pulmonary artery. In the lungs, the blood picks up oxygen that you have breathed in, and delivers carbon dioxide to be exhaled when you breathe out.

Just past the aortic valve in the aorta are the openings for the coronary arteries that supply blood to the myocardium. During systole, the open aortic valve covers these coronary entrances, but when the valve closes during the resting phase of the cycle, called diastole (pronounced "die-ass-tuh-lee"), the blood in the aorta fills the coronaries. The two coronary openings lead to the right and left coronary arteries. The left main coronary artery immediately branches into two (the circumflex toward the back of the heart and the left anterior descending toward the front). They all then go on to have many branches that interconnect with each other and supply the entire myocardium, plus there is some supply to the inside of the heart directly from the blood in the chambers.

Myocardium
The muscle tissue of the heart, similar to other muscles but contracting independently and regularly.

The entire heart is covered by a connective tissue sac called the pericardium. The lining cells inside the heart are called the endocardium, and these cells also cover the heart valves.

Arteries and Veins

The arteries are the channels that supply blood from the heart to the tissues. The veins return blood to the heart. The arteries start with the aorta, and then branch out and become smaller until they become small arterioles and then a vast network of microscopic capillaries and venules that transfer oxygen and nutrients to the tissues and remove waste. The venules start the return journey of the blood to the heart, joining with each other like small rivulets converging, and becoming larger as they get closer to the heart until they form the superior vena cava (returning from the head) and the inferior vena cava (bringing blood back from the rest of the body). The cells that line the arteries and veins are similar to those lining the heart and valves, and are called endothelial cells, or simply the endothelium.

The arteries also have connective tissue in the wall and muscle that causes the blood vessel to constrict or expand. Spasm of these muscles can constrict the vessels and cause symptoms. When the arterial endothelial cells function normally, they produce nitric oxide, also called endothelial-derived relaxing factor, a substance that causes the vessels to relax, opening up the blood flow. Nitric oxide is produced from the amino acid arginine.

Blood Pressure

When the heart pumps, sending blood into the arteries at some force, it increases the pressure inside the arterial system. The force of the blood in the arteries during the left ventricle contraction is called the systolic pressure. When the contraction ends, the pressure during the relaxation phase declines, and this is called the diastolic pressure. You will see readings of the systolic pressure over the diastolic

Systolic/ Diastolic

These terms refer to the pressure in the arteries during the contraction phase of the heart cycle (systolic) and the relaxation phase (diastolic).

pressure, such as 120/80 (read as 120 over 80). The normal range of blood pressure is from 100/60 to 120/80. In the long run, mildly elevated levels of blood pressure lead to heart and circulatory problems. In the short term, extremely high blood pressures can cause acute problems, such as headaches and strokes.

Normal pressure in the arteries is maintained by a complex interaction of hormones, sensors in the arteries, and regulatory substances involving the kidneys, the brain, and the adrenal glands. Other factors also play a role in blood pressure, including stress, physical activity, the condition of the arteries (if the arteries are stiffened by arteriosclerosis, the pressure in the system can rise), endothelial cell function, and diet.

The Electrocardiogram (EKG)

One of the most common measures of heart function is the electrocardiogram, usually abbreviated as EKG. This test evaluates the electrical activity of the heart, and creates a tracing that a doctor can use to understand the heart rhythm, learn whether the heart muscle has been damaged by a recent or past heart attack, examine the strength of the heart muscle, and other signs of heart function. Although more sophisticated tests are available (echocardiograms, stress tests, PET scans, angiograms, and others), this is one of the most basic, and it is not invasive. The EKG can be used to show improvements in heart function with treatment, or declines of function as a result of worsening disease.

CHAPTER 2

ABNORMALITIES OF THE HEART

Although the heart is a remarkable organ that usually performs consistently, it is subject to a number of potential problems with its anatomy and function. As a result, heart disease is the number-one killer in the United States and other developed countries. While genetic influences and external toxic exposures may lead to a tendency toward abnormal heart function, most heart problems are primarily related to lifestyle choices that are within your control. These include eating a healthy diet, getting regular exercise, developing positive feelings and attitudes, doing some form of stress management, avoiding toxins, and taking dietary supplements. If you make the right choices you can prevent and even treat most heart diseases and avoid the complications that they cause, while at the same time you can feel better and lead a longer, healthier life.

Arteriosclerosis

Hardening of the arteries is a process of anatomical change in the blood vessels, including damage to the lining cells called endothelium, chronic inflammatory repair activity, fatty deposits in the wall of the vessel, calcification of the wall, and narrowing of the channel, leading to eventual obstruction of blood flow to the vital organs. The material deposited in the walls of

Arteriosclerosis
Hardening of the arteries leading to obstruction of blood flow to vital organs, usually due to deposits of fatty and inflammatory substances, as a result of free-radical damage.

arteries, a combination of fat, cholesterol, inflamma-tory cells, fibrous tissue, and calcium, is known as plaque. Although other forms of damage can cause hardening of the arteries, it is usual for fatty deposits to appear in the early stages of the disease, and ath-erosclerosis refers to hardening of the arteries relat-ed to the fatty deposits.

When the narrowed arteries are those that supply the heart—the coronary arteries—the disease may cause symptoms from lack of oxygen to the heart muscle, and if the lack of oxygen persists it leads to the death of heart muscle cells. If enough heart-muscle cells are damaged, the heart might cease to function—a cardiac arrest—but most of the time only some cells are damaged. As with other arteries, the coronary arteries constrict or relax under differing conditions.

Because blood vessels are in a dynamic state of change, symptoms can come and go while the plaque in the arteries remains unchanged. However, the plaque can also change with conditions that lead to rupture of the plaque or hemorrhage into the plaque. Disruption of the plaque may be the mecha-nism leading to acute heart attacks.

The symptoms of coronary atherosclerosis in-clude shortness of breath, chest pain or pressure (or variations of this felt as pain in the shoulder, left arm, jaw, back, or wrist), weakness, palpitations, faint-ness, dizziness, or lightheadedness. The chest pain is commonly referred to as "angina pectoris"; it is sometimes described not as pain, but as a crushing sensation in the chest, and it is sometimes mistaken for indigestion.

Hypertension

Although hypertension is not specifically a disease of the heart, it increases the risk of atherosclerosis, and leads to other forms of heart disease. Hypertension, commonly known as high blood pressure, occurs when either the systolic or the diastolic pressure rises above normal while resting and remains there for a period of time. Typically it is considered a problem when the upper number (systolic pressure) rises above 140 and when the lower number (diastolic pressure) rises above 85 (the number refers to millimeters of mercury, or the pressure needed to raise a column of mercury a certain height). However, evidence indicates that even diastolic pressures below 85, but above the normal limit of 80, increase long-term health risks for strokes and hardening of the arteries.

Most of the time, high blood pressure does not lead to any symptoms unless the pressure is markedly elevated. The lack of symptoms has led to hypertension being called the "silent killer." Sometimes when a person's blood pressure is measured as high in a doctor's office, but is not high when they take it at home, even if their blood pressure machine is reasonably accurate. This phenomenon often results from the stressful feelings some people have when a doctor is testing them, and it is called "white-coat syndrome." This condition may not be benign, because such people may well routinely respond to stress with blood pressure elevation. Those who fail to recognize that their blood pressure, although normal at home, may rise in stressful situations are putting themselves at increased risk.

When the blood pressure is quite high, it may cause headaches and a sense of pressure and awareness of the heartbeat. Very high blood pressure must be treated urgently, as uncontrolled pressure at such levels can cause a stroke. Most blood pressure elevations are not in the range requiring emergency treatment, but if you have a persistent headache you should be evaluated by a doctor.

Valvular Disease

It sometimes happens that the valves that prevent backflow of blood into different chambers of the heart are defective as a result of malformation from birth or damage during life. While valve disease presents a mechanical problem that is little influenced by lifestyle habits and nutrition, the resulting abnormalities of heart function may well be helped by changes in diet, exercise, and appropriate dietary supplementation.

Aortic Valve
A tissue valve with three leaflets that separates the left ventricle from the aorta, and prevents backflow into the ventricle during the heart rest phase between contractions.

In addition to congenital malformations, heart valves can be affected by infection and calcification, both of which can impair normal function. One potential valve problem is prolapse, in which the valve leaflets are malformed or connections that hold the leaflets in place are defective. The valve may then bulge back into the heart chamber, allowing backflow of blood. Leaky valves increase the work of the heart, and may eventually lead to heart failure and related symptoms.

Backflow of blood is only one of the valve problems that can occur. They can also become closed off by thickening and calcification of the leaflets, called "stenosis." When abnormally thickened valves obstruct blood flow, circulation to the heart, the brain, and other organs is compromised. It also puts strain on the heart muscle, and in more severe cases can lead to sudden death.

Congestive Heart Failure

The left ventricle normally pumps out about 60 to 70 percent of the blood in the chamber at the beginning of systole. This percentage is called the "ejection fraction," and it reflects the functional capacity of the heart muscle. With decline of the heart muscle function, the ventricular ejection fraction goes down. Disease of the heart muscle can be from hardening of the arteries, valvular disease or hypertension causing chronic strain on the muscle, or inflammatory conditions, such as viral infections or toxic exposures.

As the decline of the left ventricle progresses, fluids back up in the blood vessels. The extra back-pressure in the system leads to fluid congestion in the lungs, causing shortness of breath. If the right ventricle is not functioning well, the fluid accumulates in the legs and liver, and is seen visibly as swelling of the ankles (edema) and moving higher in the body as the disease progresses. This combination of dysfunction and symptoms is called congestive heart failure. It does not mean that the heart has ceased to function, as in a cardiac arrest.

Congestive heart failure is a treatable condition, and with proper care and good health habits a person with congestive heart failure can function well. One of the primary medications for congestive heart failure, digitalis, has been in use for centuries if not longer, and is derived from the common garden plant, foxglove. Dietary supplements can also help treat congestive heart

Congestive Heart Failure
Inability of the heart to pump out the normal amount of blood with each beat, as a result of weakness of the heart muscle.

failure. If the condition is severe, a surgeon can implant a cardiac assist device to aid the heart muscle pumping action. In the most severe cases the only solution is a heart transplant, but that is a late-stage solution.

Arrhythmias

The rhythm of the heartbeat is controlled by a variety of electrical mechanisms in the heart muscle of both the left atrium and the left ventricle. Normally the rhythm is quite regular, although sometimes an extra beat occurs and sometimes a beat is missed without it signifying any pathology. However, if the heartbeat is persistently irregular, or extra beats are frequent, it is called a cardiac arrhythmia, and it requires treatment.

Sometimes arrhythmias cause no symptoms, but at other times they can cause palpitations (sensing a strong heartbeat, or feeling as though the heart is "jumpy"), or even shortness of breath and anxiety. Irregular heartbeats can be quite varied, including tachycardia (a very rapid heartbeat), atrial fibrillation (when the heartbeat is irregular with no particular pattern), or a consistently irregular beat.

CHAPTER 3

RISK FACTORS
FOR HEART DISEASE

Some people are more prone to develop heart disease than others. It is possible to evaluate the risk of someone developing heart disease by looking at different health habits, laboratory tests, medical history, family history, current health status, and other measures that relate to the disease. While genetic makeup plays a role, it is only one of many contributors. The following information may help you determine just how careful you have to be, but even with few risk factors, it is important to take good care of yourself, as these factors (other than genetics) may change over time.

Family History

People who have family members with heart disease are at a statistically higher risk of developing the problem themselves. However, family members often have similar health habits, so it is not at all clear that the entire familial risk is due to genetics. Nevertheless, it is likely that some genetic propensity contributes to the risk of heart disease, higher cholesterol levels, hypertension, diabetes, and strokes.

If any of your family members have heart disease or have died as a result of it, you would be well advised to make the lifestyle changes and take the dietary supplements that help prevent it. You cannot change your genetics, just as you cannot stop the inevitable advance of years, so in practical terms it is not worth worrying about aging and genetics as risk factors when you could be expending your energy in modifying those risks over which you have great influence.

Obesity

One of the risk factors for heart disease is being overweight. Carrying extra weight puts more strain on the heart and circulatory system. Obesity is a strong risk factor for developing congestive heart failure, independent of other risk factors. A modest increase in Body Mass Index (BMI, an indicator of overweight) can double the risk of coronary artery disease and other heart diseases, and the heaviest people are at an even greater risk.

Losing weight through a healthy diet and exercise program that you can keep up for the rest of your life is a highly effective way to reduce your risk of cardiac disease. Even if you do not reduce your weight to normal, any improvement in fitness through regular exercise can reduce your risk. Reducing weight is also important for controlling blood pressure, lowering blood lipids, including cholesterol and triglycerides, raising the good HDL cholesterol, and reducing resistance to blood flow in the coronaries and other arteries.

Diet

Diet plays such an important role in preventing chronic degenerative diseases, including heart disease, that I have reserved a special section for it later in the book. Although controversy still runs through the medical community, most of the scientific literature suggests that diets high in fat (particularly saturated fat, burned fat, and partially hydrogenated vegetable oils), meats, sugar and white flour (refined carbohydrates), and other highly processed foods all contribute to increased risk of heart disease.

On the other hand, diets high in vegetables, fruits, whole grains, legumes, seeds, and nuts, as well as fish (particularly oily fish, such as salmon and sardines) all contribute to reducing the risk of developing heart disease (and help to treat the disease if you already have it). Numerous fad diets have appeared in the popular press with little or no scientific justification for their purported value.

Some of the authors of health-related books and articles often seem more interested in selling those books or newsletters than in helping people become healthier. They may make outlandish claims, such as saying that all carbohydrates are bad for you (refusing to acknowledge the difference between refined carbohydrates and whole, natural foods), or mislead you into thinking that a "Paleolithic" diet has some relevance for modern humans (supporting an unhealthy high-meat or high-protein diet). It is best to avoid getting caught up in hyperbolic claims that do not include long-term studies supporting the healthy end-result you are seeking.

Sedentary Lifestyle

Being a couch potato will ruin your health in many ways, and one of them is by increasing your risk of heart disease. On the other hand, being physically active will prevent and reverse many of the changes that lead to heart disease (as well as cancer, diabetes, and other illnesses). Regular aerobic exercise reduces weight, lowers cholesterol, increases the good HDL-cholesterol, improves circulation, lowers blood pressure, enhances insulin sensitivity, and makes you feel good while increasing your energy. This is definitely one risk factor over which you have control, and almost any form of activity is helpful.

While it is good to have a regular exercise program, it is also valuable to be physically active in your daily living habits—taking stairs instead of elevators, walking to the post office instead of driving, walking a dog, gardening, bicycling on errands, and doing housework. All of these activities contribute to your fitness and reduce your heart-disease risks.

Smoking

Tobacco use, whether smoking or chewing tobacco, increases the risk of heart disease more than any other risk factor. Cigarettes cause the most increase in risk, but cigars and pipes are also contributors to risk, as is secondhand smoke. Giving up smoking is probably the most effective way to reduce your heart disease risk. Tobacco smoke is one of the greatest sources of free radicals, highly damaging chemicals that lead to arterial damage, and also lead to increased risk of cancer.

Hypertension

While this is a condition rather than a lifestyle choice, high blood pressure is another risk factor for the development of atherosclerotic heart disease. Any blood pressure over 120/80 leads to an increase of risk of atherosclerosis (as previously discussed). While it is not always possible to control blood pressure without medications, most of the time diet and other lifestyle changes, as well as dietary supplements, can reduce or eliminate the need for medical therapy.

Insulin Resistance

Insulin is a hormone produced in the pancreas that controls the level of blood sugar (glucose). Insulin is needed to allow glucose to pass into cells so they can use it to produce energy. Most cells require insulin, including muscle cells, but insulin is not needed for glucose to pass into brain cells, where it is a critical fuel. The situation is complicated by the variation in the cells' ability to respond to insulin. In certain circumstances, the cells become resistant to the effects of insulin. If cells are less sensitive to insulin, the pancreas compensates by increasing insulin production resulting in a number of subsequent effects.

Insulin resistance syndrome (also called Syndrome X, or metabolic syndrome) is a collection of abnormalities including excess insulin production, diabetes, obesity, blood fat abnormalities (low HDL levels and high triglycerides), hypertension, and heart disease.

However, it is not clear that any of these conditions are themselves caused by the insulin resistance, except that high levels of insulin may well be related to atherosclerotic damage to the arteries.

The most likely cause of insulin resistance is a combination of being overweight and lack of exercise, both of which lead to the abnormalities associated with the condition. Insulin resistance itself can lead to a further increase in obesity, as the excess insulin in the blood triggers the brain to crave more food, and the liver to create more fat. In other words, insulin resistance may be the result of the conditions associated with the syndrome, rather than the cause, even though insulin itself is damaging to tissues.

The best treatments for insulin resistance are exercise and diet, although not the high-protein diets that are often recommended. Complex carbohydrates, such as those found in whole grains, legumes, and vegetables, are beneficial to people with insulin resistance, while refined grains (white flour, white rice, and refined corn, for examples) and sugar (as found in sweets and other desserts) are damaging, and make insulin resistance worse (see the "glycemic index" in the diet section). Appropriate dietary supplements can also help control blood sugar, increase insulin sensitivity, and reduce many of the risk factors associated with the insulin resistance syndrome.

Alcohol Consumption

Heart disease risk is lower in France than in the United States. However, it is still the number-one cause of death in France, and wine consumption does not offer consistent protection. A moderate amount of alcohol of any kind, including red wine, may offer some protection, but excessive alcohol consumption increases heart disease risk. Too much alcohol can increase blood pressure and damage the heart muscle, increasing the risk of heart failure.

Stress

High stress levels, or the perception of being under high stress, contribute to heart disease. Stress can raise blood pressure, constrict arteries, precipitate arrhythmias of the heart, and have other damaging effects. If someone already has atherosclerosis, stress might precipitate spasms of the coronary arteries and lead to a heart attack. Stress can make congestive heart failure worse, and heart patients have a higher mortality if they are under emotional stress and are anxious or depressed. Stress also affects hormone levels, regulatory messengers called prostaglandins, and inflammatory substances in the blood and tissues.

Stress may make it difficult to follow healthy eating and exercise habits. This makes it all the more important to develop healthy habits before stressful events make it more difficult. The more ingrained such habits are, the easier it is to follow them when something stressful does occur. It is also helpful to learn stress-reduction habits so that in difficult times you are able to draw on these previously developed methods of coping.

Diabetes

People with diabetes have higher rates of heart disease. If their blood sugar is not under control, the risk is even higher, but even diabetics with relatively good sugar control are at increased risk of coronary artery disease. Most diabetics have adult onset, or type 2, diabetes (as opposed to type 1, or juvenile diabetes). While type 1 diabetes can be influenced by lifestyle changes, type 2 diabetes is almost completely preventable by lifestyle changes, and it can often be treated and reversed through weight control, diet, exercise, and a variety of dietary supplements.

Dental Disease (Periodontal Disease)

A number of studies now show that chronic inflammation of the gums (gingivitis, or periodontitis) is associated with an increased risk of heart disease. Periodontitis is due to a chronic bacterial infection of the gums. As a result, bacterial and inflammatory byproducts are absorbed into the blood. This chronic condition is associated with an increase of the blood level of C-reactive protein (CRP; discussed below), and an increase in heart disease. Severe periodontitis, or loss of teeth due to gum disease, doubles the risk. It is apparent that chronic inflammation or low-grade infection of any kind may contribute to heart risk, possibly due to the production of free radicals (see below), as well as the increase in CRP.

Other Risk Factors

Hormone imbalances, long-term birth control pill use (mainly in smokers), low thyroid function, declining testosterone and estrogen levels with age, and age-related loss of growth-hormone production are all contributors to heart disease risk. In addition, heavy metal exposure can increase the risk of heart disease. This is a particular problem with mercury excess that comes from eating too much contaminated fish, such as swordfish, shark, and tuna, from mercury amalgam in dental fillings, immunization with mercury-preserved vaccines, and environmental exposures.

In women, hormone therapy with conjugated estrogens (Premarin) and medroxyprogesterone (Provera) was thought to reduce the risk of heart disease, but recent clinical trials suggest the opposite, and the use of these hormones has dropped off considerably. Using natural hormones that are identical to human hormone profiles are more likely to provide benefits without the same risks. Growth-hormone therapy may also provide benefits for the aging population, including restoration of heart muscle function.

Blood Tests Indicating
Heart Disease Risks

In addition to lifestyle, genetics, and health conditions, various blood tests can indicate the risk of heart disease. If you know the results of these tests, you can take certain steps to change them through diet, supplements, or other health habits.

Cholesterol

Although the blood level of cholesterol is related to the risk of developing heart disease, it is not as important as many other risk factors in both lifestyle and in laboratory tests. People with serum cholesterol under 150 milligrams/deciliter virtually never get heart disease. Higher levels of cholesterol are associated with increasing risk, but it is not clear that lowering cholesterol through drug therapy is beneficial for everyone.

High-density lipoprotein cholesterol (HDL) is known as the good cholesterol because its smaller particles are more easily cleared from the system. The ratio of total cholesterol to HDL is often used as a marker for "cardiac risk" in laboratory reports. Lower ratios are associated with lower risk. The average ratio is 5 to 1 for men, and 3 to 1 or lower is associated with half the risk. The averages are lower for women.

LDL, or low-density lipoprotein cholesterol, is the damaging form of cholesterol; the oxidized form of LDL is most damaging. Oxidation of LDL can be modified with diet and dietary supplements.

Homocysteine

Homocysteine is a sulfur-containing amino acid in the blood, related to methionine. The amount of homocysteine in the blood is higher with lower levels of folic acid, vitamin B_{12}, and vitamin B_6, as well as other nutrients. High levels of homocysteine are related to an increased risk of cardiovascular disease and brain degeneration as seen in Alzheimer's disease (the higher levels of homocysteine can double this risk). People with the highest levels of homocysteine had 2.2 times the risk for cardiovascular disease as people with the lowest levels.

Homocysteine levels as a risk factor for vascular

disease were first demonstrated over thirty years ago. At that time the doctor who wrote about it, Dr. Kilmer McCully, was denigrated by his colleagues, but he has since been vindicated and his theories accepted. Dietary supplements can significantly lower levels of homocysteine, reducing the risk of heart disease, cerebral vascular disease, and Alzheimer's disease.

C-Reactive Protein (CRP)

C-reactive protein (CRP) is a protein produced in the liver, and the amount in the blood is a nonspecific marker for inflammation. The higher the CRP, the more likely it is that someone has inflammation somewhere in the body. In recent years, it has become clear that using a highly sensitive test for CRP (hs-CRP) is useful as an indicator of heart disease risk. People with the highest levels of CRP have seven times the risk of having a heart attack or stroke compared to those people with the lowest levels. Elevated CRP levels are more predictive of heart disease than cholesterol levels. People with subclinical infections with certain bacteria appear to be at higher risk of cardiovascular disease.

CRP may be more than a marker, as some evidence suggests that it can itself cause inflammation of the arterial wall, increasing the risk that plaque will rupture and cause a heart attack. Oral contraceptive use can elevate CRP levels, and the common estrogen treatment with Premarin (estrogens from pregnant horses) can raise CRP levels by 64 percent after twelve months of treatment. CRP levels are higher in obese people, particularly if they are insulin resistant, while weight loss can significantly lower CRP levels.

A Note on Free Radicals

While not a specific risk factor, free radicals play a role in the development of many degenerative diseases, including heart disease. In the normal course of metabolism, your body produces small high-energy particles called free radicals. These are molecules with free electrons that can be channeled into energy production. In some cells they may be used as the weapons to kill viruses and bacteria. Because of their extremely high energy, free radicals can also be highly damaging to normal tissues. If too many free radicals are produced, or if we are exposed to them from external sources, they can overwhelm the protective systems, which consist of enzymes and vitamins.

Free Radicals
High energy molecules that are not stable because they lack an electron, and do damage to cells and tissues while finding that lost electron. Most damaging free radicals are related to oxygen.

Most of the free radicals are related to oxygen, and they lead to oxidative damage to genes (disrupting the normal production of DNA and RNA), cell membranes, and lipids. They also damage the endothelium in the heart and blood vessels, and they distort the production of prostaglandins, which regulate many physiological functions.

Free radicals are also found in the environment. There are many sources of excess free radicals, including toxic metals, cigarette smoke, air pollution, many drugs, highly processed foods and food additives, ultraviolet sunlight, and radiation.

By careful lifestyle choices, you can avoid many of these free-radical sources and you can protect yourself from others. By making these choices for yourself you can slow down the aging process, while decreasing the risk of cancer and heart disease.

CHAPTER 4

BASIC NUTRITIONAL SUPPLEMENTS FOR THE HEART

Numerous dietary supplements help to both prevent and treat heart diseases, and they work especially well when combined with a comprehensive health program of diet, exercise, relaxation, and other natural therapies. Supplements help to improve the risk factors for heart disease, such as total and HDL cholesterol levels in the serum, homocysteine levels, and the inflammatory marker CRP. They can help control blood pressure, spasm of coronary arteries, inflammation, excessive platelet aggregation, and heart rhythm.

Supplements can also reduce oxidation of LDL and other sources of free-radical damage to lipids, cell membranes, and DNA. Some dietary supplements are also important contributors to the reversal of insulin resistance and the syndrome associated with it. In fact, in addition to other lifestyle changes, including diet, exercise, relaxation, and stress reduction, dietary supplements can modify virtually every risk factor for cardiovascular disease, and they may replace drugs as treatment for many conditions. However, for some conditions they may not work as quickly or as dramatically as drugs (although they avoid the side effects), and combinations of supplements may be essential to achieve the benefits. Sometimes they are helpful if they are used in conjunction with medications, at least until the condition is under control, at which time it may be possible to eliminate the medications while continuing the safer dietary supplements.

B Vitamins

Among a variety of dietary supplements, the B vitamins are commonly grouped together because of physiological or biochemical similarities. Several of them have value in preventing and treating heart disease, and modifying the known risk factors.

Cobalamin (Vitamin B$_{12}$)

Vitamin B$_{12}$ is an essential nutrient for normal red blood cell formation, DNA production, and the development and maintenance of the brain and nerve tissue. Deficiency of B$_{12}$ in the early stages causes anemia, and chronic deficiency leads to nerve degeneration. Supplements are often beneficial to elderly people with depression and fatigue, sometimes requiring high doses. In addition, B$_{12}$ is one of the nutrients that help to lower serum levels of homocysteine, the risk factor for heart disease, along with vitamin B$_6$ and folic acid.

People with high homocysteine levels are very likely to have low levels of vitamin B$_{12}$ in their blood and tissues. Absorption of vitamin B$_{12}$ from the intestinal tract, requires hydrochloric acid from the stomach digestive juices, as well as a substance called "intrinsic factor" that is also produced in the stomach lining. The B$_{12}$ is actually absorbed through the tissues that line the end of the small intestine, or ileum. With age, production of hydrochloric acid declines, and if the stomach lining degenerates (atrophies) the production of intrinsic factor goes down. Other people who might not absorb B$_{12}$ are those with inflammatory diseases of the small intestine, such as Crohn's disease. Because oral B$_{12}$ may not be well absorbed, some elderly patients benefit from injections of this vitamin.

In the diet, the most reliable sources of vitamin B$_{12}$ are eggs, fish, milk, and meats, of which, the healthiest sources are eggs and fish. Research shows that B$_{12}$ is also present in a bioavailable form in some seaweed (nori, or laver), which may be a valuable source for people on vegan diets (strict vegetarians who eat no animal products at all). Common forms of B_{12} include cyano-cobalamin, hydroxo-cobalamin, and methyl-cobalamin, and supplements of each are available. Typical oral doses of B_{12} range from 1,000 micrograms (1 mg) up to 5,000 micrograms (5 mg) per day. Such high doses help to force B_{12} across the intestinal membrane to make up for poor absorption.

Folic Acid

Folic acid (also known as folate) is a B vitamin that is essential for red blood cell and DNA formation, as well as for growth and division of cells and for the manufacture of protein. Food sources of folate include leafy greens (the name comes from "foliage"), beans, whole grains, and citrus fruits. In the growing fetus, folate is essential for neurological development, and deficiency leads to congenital malformations including failure of brain formation (anencephaly), incomplete closure of the spine (spina bifida, a neural tube defect), and other neurological and organ abnormalities. Deficiency of folic acid also causes one form of anemia.

Folic acid in food or in supplements can help prevent birth defects, but most of the research suggests that supplements are the more reliable source. Folic acid may also be important in reducing the risk of cancer of the breast, colon, pancreas, and lung. It is one of the nutrients that help to lower the serum level of homocysteine, thus reducing the risk of cardiovascular disease.

The usual dose of folic acid in supplements is 100 to 400 micrograms, and for pregnancy 800 micrograms is commonly prescribed. However, evidence is mounting that higher levels are valuable in reducing a number of health risks, including heart disease, and doses as high as 5,000 to 20,000 micrograms (5 to 20 mg) can more effectively lower homocysteine than the usual supplements. Folic acid is available from some vitamin companies in doses of 5,000 micrograms (5 mg) or more.

Niacin (Vitamin B₃)

Niacin (also called nicotinic acid), or vitamin B_3, is essential for healthy skin, intestinal function, and mental function. Your body needs niacin to process carbohydrates into energy, and for protein and fat metabolism, and it is also required to metabolize alcohol. Food sources include whole grains, peanuts and other legumes, nuts, seeds, and vegetables, as well as meats. A deficiency of niacin causes pellagra, a condition with varied symptoms including mental illness, skin disorders, and digestive disturbances. The therapeutic levels needed for heart disease protection are much higher than you can get from food.

Supplements of niacin in high doses have been used for years as a cholesterol-lowering treatment, although such doses may have some side effects. The most prominent unwanted effect is a flush of the skin that lasts for about twenty to sixty minutes and is due to a sudden release of histamine. This can be uncomfortable, with redness and itching, and in a few people it can be severe. The flush can be reduced by taking timed-release niacin. It is also possible to have abnormal liver-function tests from taking niacin in large daily doses over time, and with the timed-release form even hepatitis, although this is rare.

A nonflush form of niacin, inositol hexaniacinate, is also available. It is effective in reducing cholesterol, and has most of the other desired effects of niacin. Another form of vitamin B_3, niacinamide (or nicotinamide), does not cause flushing or have negative effects on the liver, but while it is useful for treating B_3 deficiency and some forms of mental illness, it is not effective in lowering cholesterol, and preventing heart disease.

A report in 2002 showed that in diabetics, high doses of niacin could reduce the risk of a second heart attack by 50 percent (even though the niacin slightly raised their blood sugar levels). The treatment led to lower cholesterol, LDL cholesterol, and triglyceride levels, while raising the good HDL cholesterol, and it is thought to have other beneficial effects. This result was equal to the other treatments for preventing heart attacks, including statin drugs, aspirin, and beta-blockers, but without their side effects (statins reduce production of coenzyme Q_{10} and can cause muscle damage; aspirin can cause gastrointestinal bleeding and kidney disease; and beta-blockers can cause fatigue, depression, sexual dysfunction, and weakness).

In other reports, taking 3,000 milligrams of niacin daily has lowered heart attack risk by 28 percent over a six-year period in people without diabetes, and over fifteen years, the risk of dying of heart disease was cut by 11 percent. A review in 2003 showed that niacin was the most effective single therapy to raise HDL and reduce harmful lipids, including LDL, and to reduce heart disease and mortality, and it did not lead to adverse interactions with any other therapy.

Niacin also decreases the level of another heart disease risk factor called lipoprotein (a), or Lp(a), while none of the prescription medications have that effect. It not only prevents heart disease and its progression in patients who already have the condition, but also promotes regression of atherosclerotic plaques. Niacin has some anti-inflammatory effects, and it helps to stabilize plaque (unstable plaque is one cause of heart attacks).

For heart patients, or for those with elevated cholesterol and triglyceride levels, typical recommended daily doses of niacin are from 1,500 to 3,000 milligrams. Taking timed release niacin will usually reduce or eliminate the flushing reaction. Inositol hexaniacinate eliminates the concern about the flush, and appears to have the same benefits without any apparent risks to the liver. It is possible that with combinations of other dietary supplements the dose of niacin can be reduced while still achieving the same benefits.

Pyridoxine (Vitamin B₆)

Pyridoxine, or vitamin B_6, is essential for metabolism of proteins, fats, and carbohydrates, and it participates in the production of some hormones. It is also involved in the production of red blood cells, and it supports normal immune function. Low intake of pyridoxine contributes to an increase in homocysteine levels, raising the risk of heart disease, while supplements, along with folic acid and vitamin B_{12}, can reduce levels of this cardiac risk factor.

Supplements of pyridoxine can reduce nausea and vomiting associated with pregnancy, enhance immune function, lessen symptoms of PMS, and treat carpal tunnel syndrome. In addition, pyridoxine has been used for treatment of a variety of mental disorders, including depression and Attention Deficit Disorder (ADD). Some people who have taken very high doses of pyridoxine for months have developed neuropathy in the extremities, with symptoms of numbness and tingling, and weakness in the arms and legs. This is not common, and the doses associated with problems were in the range of 2,000 to 6,000 milligrams daily for six to nine months. Pyridoxine is valuable in doses of 50 to 200 milligrams, and in some situations even higher doses may be helpful in lowering homocysteine levels.

Vitamin C

Vitamin C, or ascorbic acid, is an essential nutrient with a broad range of functions in human metabolism. Only a few animals do not make their own vitamin C, including humans and other primates, guinea pigs, and fish, and they must consume vitamin C in the diet or as supplements to avoid the deficiency disease known as scurvy. The best dietary sources of vitamin C are citrus fruits, black currants, berries, broccoli and other cabbage family vegetables, and potatoes, but it is destroyed by cooking or long-term storage at room temperature.

Vitamin C became popular in the 1970s after Linus Pauling, Ph.D., a world-renowned chemist and two-time Nobel Prize winner, wrote a book on the value of very-high-dose vitamin C for colds and flu infections. However, vitamin C had been used in high doses by some physicians since the 1940s, and for far more than colds. Although controversial, the weight of evidence suggests that vitamin C is beneficial in treating infectious diseases, and even high doses are without serious side effects.

Vitamin C is a potent antioxidant, protecting tissues from free-radical damage. It works with vitamin E to prevent these dangerous reactions from getting out of control. Vitamin C is essential for the production of collagen, the base substance that forms connective tissue, as well as for neurotransmitter and hormone production. It also helps the absorption of iron in the gastrointestinal tract. Vitamin C is essential for immune function, resistance to infection, and white blood cell activity. It also helps the enzymes that metabolize drugs and toxins.

Deficiency of vitamin C leads to bruising and bleeding, deterioration of the gums, loose teeth, and impaired wound healing, all the signs of scurvy. One of the earliest signs of vitamin C deficiency is fatigue. Vitamin C in high doses is helpful in cancer treatment, chronic fatigue, infections, and asthma. It also increases bone density, improves surgical outcomes, helps fight stress, and enhances healing from burns.

Vitamin C also has some functions that are specific for heart and vascular health. It protects the endothelium to promote the production of nitric oxide (the blood vessel relaxing factor), and can lower blood pressure while it promotes arterial health. In a study of hypertension, patients were given 500 milligrams of vitamin C daily, and were monitored for blood pressure changes for three months. Blood pressures were moderately reduced, and at the same time lipid levels were improved. Another study showed that 2,000 milligrams of vitamin C daily could improve the function of blood vessels, helping them to relax and enhance blood flow. Intravenous vitamin C protects endothelium from tobacco smoke oxidative damage.

In congestive heart failure, vitamin C can protect the heart muscle cells, particularly when the heart rhythm is abnormal. It also helps with insulin resistance. A study of both smokers and nonsmokers showed that vitamin C improved their endothelial function, and if they had abnormal sugar regulation, the vitamin C enhanced their insulin sensitivity.

Vitamin C inhibits the excessive aggregation of platelets, resulting in decreased risk of blood clots forming in the arteries and obstructing blood flow to the heart. In one study, subjects were given 3,000 milligrams of vitamin C intravenously and monitored for platelet activity. Within six hours, and for up to twenty-four hours, the vitamin C supplements were effective in reducing platelet aggregation. The authors of this study concluded that the vitamin provided a protective effect against the development of coronary heart disease. In smokers, those with the highest intake of vitamin C have only 34 percent the risk of developing heart disease as those with the lowest intake. (Non-smokers with high vitamin C intake fared even better.)

In the large Nurses' Health Study, started in 1980 at Harvard University, researchers found that vitamin C intake was directly related to a reduced risk of heart disease and mortality. They studied 85,000 subjects over sixteen years and noted that those in the highest category of vitamin C intake had a 27 percent lower risk of mortality from heart disease. When they removed those who took supplements from their calculations, the variation from diet alone showed no significant difference. To quote the authors, "Among women who did not use vitamin C supplements or multivitamins, the association between intake of vitamin C from diet alone and incidence of heart disease was weak and not significant." This means that it is the supplement takers who get real benefits from vitamin C.

Typical doses of vitamin C supplements can vary widely. A basic amount in supplements is often 200 to 500 milligrams, but much higher doses may be beneficial for a wide range of conditions. It may well be beneficial to take 2,000 to 6,000 milligrams daily for protection against heart disease, cancer, and hypertension.

Vitamin E

Vitamin E is a fat-soluble nutrient found in nuts, seeds, unprocessed vegetable oils, whole grains, beans, and green vegetables. It is a potent biological antioxidant that works with vitamin C, and it protects cell membrane fatty acids from oxygen free-radical damage. Even with a healthy diet, it is not possible to consume the levels of vitamin E that have been shown to be beneficial. Supplements are the most reliable way to get adequate therapeutic levels of this vitamin.

Vitamin E is necessary for development of nerves and muscles, and for maintenance of their function, and it helps prevent cataract formation. People with high levels of vitamin E in the blood are at a lower risk of developing macular degeneration, an eye disorder associated with aging and oxidative damage. High doses of vitamin E can enhance immunity, reduce platelet aggregation, and improve the lipid levels in the blood. It is very likely that high doses of vitamin E can reduce heart disease risks and recurrence of heart attacks in people who already have heart disease. It protects the heart muscle from damage due to rapid heart rates, a form of arrhythmia that leads to excess oxidative damage.

Although it was thought at one time that vitamin E might increase blood pressure, recent evidence shows that it has the opposite effect. In one study of seventy subjects with mild hypertension, half were given 200 IU of vitamin E per day, and the others a placebo. At the end of twenty-seven weeks, the treatment group had a 24 percent decline in systolic pressure and a 12 percent decline in diastolic pressure. There was no change in the placebo group.

Studies of vitamin E and heart disease are not consistent in their results, and it is sometimes difficult to interpret the findings. No studies show that vitamin E is harmful in heart disease, and a number of studies show that it is beneficial. The Cambridge Heart Antioxidant Study in England showed that 400 to 800 IU of vitamin E reduced the rate of recurrence of fatal and nonfatal heart attacks. Another trial showed that vitamin E had little effect on heart attack rates.

It is possible that the clinical benefits of vitamin E supplements that one would expect from its known functions (inhibition of platelets, reducing inflammation, improving lipid levels) may take years to become apparent. It may be that such benefits will only be evident in people with specific risks. Because it is very unlikely that taking vitamin E in any dose is harmful, it is a good idea to take it even though the research is still being developed, and it has many other benefits at the same time. Typical doses of vitamin E are 400 to 800 IU daily, although higher doses may also be valuable.

Magnesium

Magnesium is a particularly important mineral for maintaining healthy heart function and for treatment of a variety of heart conditions. It is a cofactor for the activity of over 300 enzymes that are essential for sugar metabolism, energy production, and protein and DNA manufacture. Magnesium is also important for the production of bone, and it is required for the transmission of nerve impulses and for muscle activity. Insulin activity also depends on magnesium.

The best dietary sources of magnesium are whole grains, leafy green vegetables (magnesium is the central atom in chlorophyll), seeds, and nuts. Oatmeal is a good source, as are potatoes (with the peel), and whole wheat (which has three times as much as white flour). Magnesium levels found in the typical diet in the United States are much too low, but inadequate magnesium is difficult to detect until it is advanced. A deficiency of magnesium leads to muscle and nerve irritability, fatigue, spasm of the blood vessel muscles (leading to high blood pressure, angina, and heart attacks). Magnesium also serves to balance calcium in tissues and cells, which otherwise tends to accumulate inside cells with age, interfering with normal enzyme functions.

Magnesium supplements help to lower blood pressure, reduce the likelihood of heart attacks due to coronary artery spasm, and control cardiac arrhythmias. A review of studies on intravenous magnesium therapy in heart attack patients showed that it reduced in-hospital mortality by 20 percent, and it reduced arrhythmias and heart failure by 25 percent. A study of over 12,000 individuals showed that mortality from heart disease was directly related to lower levels of magnesium in the serum, which was most likely due to inadequate dietary intake. Those people with the highest levels of magnesium had a 21 to 34 percent lower risk of dying of heart disease.

When patients are treated with diuretic drugs for hypertension or heart failure, it is usually understood by their physicians that the treatment might cause a deficiency of potassium, and they take measures to ensure adequate potassium intake to make up for this. What is not as well recognized is that most diuretics also deplete magnesium, and that this should also be supplemented for those patients.

Atrial fibrillation is a common arrhythmia in the elderly, particularly after heart surgery. Magnesium supplements can help reduce the incidence of this abnormality. In a study of over 200 heart surgery patients, those who were given magnesium supplements had a 60 percent reduction of atrial fibrillation compared to the placebo group (when magnesium was combined with an appropriate medication, the risk was even further reduced). Another study showed a 90 percent reduction with magnesium alone. Magnesium taken orally is also valuable for other cardiac arrhythmias.

Typical doses of magnesium range from 500 to 1,000 milligrams of elemental magnesium. Most people will absorb a significant amount of magnesium from any supplemental form, but some forms of magnesium are better absorbed than others. Among the best forms are magnesium aspartate and magnesium ascorbate. Magnesium oxide is also common in supplements, but it is not as well absorbed as some other forms. Taking magnesium with vitamin B_6 can enhance the transport of the mineral into cells.

Chromium

Chromium is an essential trace mineral that is necessary for proper blood sugar regulation. As such, it is helpful for people with hypoglycemia, a condition with fluctuating blood sugars that may cause a variety of psychological, neurological, and physiological symptoms, including fatigue, headaches, depression, irritability, palpitations, and insomnia. Chromium also helps regulate blood lipids, lowering total cholesterol and raising the good HDL cholesterol.

Chromium is found in the diet primarily in whole wheat, seeds, nuts, berries, and raisins. Sugar in the diet causes loss of chromium and an increased need for the mineral. A few studies suggest that chromium supplements might help with weight loss and muscle building, both of which would in turn assist in the prevention and treatment of heart disease. However, it is unlikely that any dietary supplement works for either weight control or bodybuilding without a complete program of diet and exercise at the same time, and long-term maintenance of healthy weight requires lifestyle changes, as well as supplements.

Because of its role in blood sugar regulation, chromium is valuable for diabetics and people with insulin resistance. Diabetics are particularly resistant to the effects of chromium, and need much higher levels than the usual dose of 200 micrograms that is recommended. In fact, type 2 diabetics respond so well to 1,000 micrograms daily that most of them are able to eliminate medications and maintain normal blood sugar levels. Diabetics on medication need to be aware that their medication needs might be reduced by supplemental chromium, causing hypo-glycemia if they do not adjust their dose.

Because of its role in controlling diabetes and helping with insulin resistance and blood lipids, chromium is valuable for prevention and treatment of heart disease. Typical doses for general health and prevention range from 100 to 400 micrograms daily, and for diabetics, the usual recommended dose is 1,000 micrograms daily. The forms of supplemental chromium that are available have some differences in their clinical effectiveness, but in general these differences are small relative to the recommended doses. Chromium picolinate, GTF chromium (GTF stands for "glucose tolerance factor"), and chromi-um polynicotinate are the most commonly available forms.

CHAPTER 5

ADVANCED NUTRITIONAL SUPPLEMENTS FOR THE HEART

The heart and blood vessels are damaged and made susceptible to disease by oxidative free radicals and by inflammation, two important contributors to heart disease risk (as well as to other chronic, degenerative diseases). Protection from both inflammation and oxygen free radicals are two of the most important parts of a preventive medicine program, and are also valuable in treatment protocols. Numerous dietary components, whether from food or supplements, contribute to this protective system. These include enzymes that your body produces, and others that are found in both food and dietary supplements. Some of these are required in the diet at all times because you never make them, and others are needed when your body production declines due to the aging process, stress, toxic exposures that interfere with metabolism, or drug side effects.

In addition to these protective supplements, other food components and supplements are required for basic metabolic functions of the heart muscle and the arteries, detoxifying cellular metabolism, and normal cellular energy production. A number of these nutrients serve more than one function (for example, they may be antioxidants and contribute to energy production, or they may be anti-inflammatory and help with detoxification).

Coenzyme Q_{10}

Coenzyme Q_{10} (CoQ_{10}) is a fat-soluble nutrient related to vitamin E, with even more potent antioxidant properties and a critical function in the production of energy in every cell, but especially in heart muscle. It is also a critical protective antioxidant in the brain. We produce coenzyme Q_{10} in normal metabolism, and it is present in foods, but only in very small amounts. Although we get some in the diet it is not adequate for health, especially as we age, when the production of CoQ_{10} declines.

The cells make energy for storage in little "engines" called mitochondria. The mitochondria have membranes, inside which energy is produced. The energy storage molecule is called ATP, and in order to make ATP the mitochondria require coenzyme Q_{10} (as well as a supply of fatty acids that are carried across the mitochondrial membranes by L-carnitine). As the heart uses a lot of energy, CoQ_{10} is particularly important for heart health, but the brain also benefits from CoQ_{10}. Recent studies show that CoQ_{10} supplements can treat Parkinson's disease and Alzheimer's disease, as well as other brain degenerative disorders. Other research shows that CoQ_{10} is also helpful in gingivitis (inflammation of the gums, or periodontal disease).

Dietary supplements of CoQ_{10} enhance immune function, help control sugar levels in diabetes, and may help reverse breast cancer if taken in high enough doses. In addition to all these extra benefits, CoQ_{10} is probably best known for its effect on the heart. It is known to treat high blood pressure, reverse congestive heart failure, reduce angina pectoris, and help with cardiac arrhythmias. After just a few months on 150 milligrams of CoQ_{10} every day, half of the hypertensive patients in one study were able to completely eliminate their use of blood pressure medications.

Some of the patients in this study also had congestive heart failure. Severity of heart failure is graded from category I to IV by the New York Heart Association. These patients averaged a 2.4 classification before treatment, but after a few months of treatment with this dose of CoQ_{10} the classification improved to an average of only 1.4. It is possible that with higher doses even more patients would have improved in both blood pressure control and heart failure grade. It is known now that in some people and in some health conditions higher doses do have extra benefits.

A study of patients after acute heart attacks showed that supplementing them with 120 milligrams daily of CoQ_{10} provided remarkable benefits. During a 28-day follow-up, the treatment group had a 65 percent reduction of angina, a 60 percent reduction of arrhythmias, and markedly better left ventricle function. In addition, second heart attacks and deaths from heart attacks were reduced by 50 percent in the treatment group.

In another treatment protocol, 100 milligrams of coenzyme Q_{10} and 500 micrograms of selenium (an antioxidant cofactor) were administered to patients who had just had an acute heart attack. The mortality after one year was much lower in the groups receiving the supplements (one out of thirty-two patients) compared to the controls (six out of twenty-nine patients). In addition, the control group had EKG evidence that ventricular function worsened during the course of the study, while the treatment group did not have these EKG changes, indicating that the treatment was effective in preserving the myocardium and reducing mortality.

Typical doses of CoQ_{10} range from 100 milligrams for prevention to 400 milligrams for a variety of heart conditions. Even higher doses may help even further; 1,200 milligrams have been given to Parkinson's patients with benefit, and the researchers who did that study are now studying even higher doses—up to 2,400 milligrams daily. As CoQ_{10} is fat soluble, it is best absorbed when mixed with some oily foods, including nut butters, seeds, or oily fish. One available form is mixed with lecithin in a chewable tablet, and this has been very effective. Others are emulsified gels that are well absorbed, but more expensive.

L-Carnitine

L-carnitine is one of many amino acids (these are
the molecules that are linked together in long chains
to form proteins), but it is not normally required in
the diet as are the eight essential amino acids. It
is derived from another amino acid in the body,
L-lysine, but has its own distinct functions. It is man-
ufactured in the liver and kidneys, so it is not considered an essential nutrient, but a small amount is
found in the diet. The amount that the liver makes
declines with age and with certain health problems.
If the amount that is necessary is higher than the
body can make, it becomes a "conditionally essential" nutrient, and supplements are needed. L-carnitine is particularly important for the muscles and
heart, primarily for the production of energy. In order
for energy to be produced by the mitochondria (see
coenzyme Q_{10} above), fatty acids must be carried
across the mitochondrial membrane. L-carnitine is
the essential substance for this membrane transport
of the fatty acids.

During episodes of angina, when the heart is not
receiving adequate oxygen, the level of L-carnitine in
the heart muscle declines rapidly. The heart muscle
cells can then not make energy from fats, so they
switch to carbohydrate as a source of fuel. This
can make the symptoms worse. Having adequate
L-carnitine in the tissues is a safeguard that helps
to assure adequate energy resources for the heart
muscle in times of oxygen deprivation.

Patients with heart muscle inflammation (cardiomyopathy) and congestive heart failure have low
levels of L-carnitine in their myocardium. A study of
thirty-eight patients with congestive heart failure,
from chronic hypertension or atherosclerotic heart
disease, showed that those given 2,000 milligrams of
L-carnitine per day had less difficulty breathing,
lower heart rates, less edema, and a reduction in
their need for medication. At the same time, the

patients felt better, and their cholesterol and triglyceride levels came down.

In another study of heart failure and atherosclerosis, patients were given 3,000 milligrams of L-carnitine daily and monitored for exercise tolerance, heart rate, blood pressure, and EKG changes suggestive of inadequate blood getting to the heart muscle. All of the measures improved with treatment compared with the placebo group over a period of 120 days. At the end of this time, the researchers stopped the treatment; they reviewed the subjects again two months later and found that the improvements had persisted even after treatment ended.

In one research protocol, patients with mild to moderate heart failure were given 1,500 milligrams of L-carnitine daily and given a stress test on a stationary bicycle. At thirty days, the amount of time they could exercise was increased significantly, and the improvement was even greater at 90 and 180 days. In these subjects, exercise time improved by 16 percent at the first test, and then 23 and 26 percent at the subsequent tests. Their ventricular ejection fractions increased by 8 percent at the first test, and then by 12 and 14 percent at the later tests. In more recent research on patients with more severe heart failure, administration of 2,000 milligrams of L-carnitine significantly reduced mortality over a three-year period.

L-carnitine also helps to reverse some cardiac arrhythmias. In patients with atherosclerotic heart disease and irregular extra heartbeats, 6 grams a day of L-carnitine significantly reduced the number of extra beats when measured with a monitor for twenty-four hours. For heart attack patients, taking 4,000 milligrams daily can reduce angina, lower blood pressure, control heart rate, and cut mortality in one year by 90 percent in a particular study. When patients with acute heart attacks were studied in a double-blind, placebo-controlled trial with 2,000 milligrams of L-carnitine, after four weeks the treatment group had a 50 percent reduction in angina, a 33 percent lower rate of severe heart failure, and half as many arrhythmias. In addition, the mortality was reduced by 40 percent with L-carnitine administration.

Typical doses of L-carnitine range from 1,000 to 6,000 milligrams daily, and it has been used in an effort to enhance athletic performance at doses up to 20,000 milligrams with no apparent side effects. In combination with other supplements and appropriate medications, L-carnitine can greatly enhance the prognosis of cardiac patients, and help them to feel better and live longer.

Essential Fatty Acids

Fats and oils play a significant and complex role in physiology and biochemistry. The essential fatty acids are those that you must consume in the diet, as the body does not make them. These polyunsaturated oils fall into two categories called omega-3 and omega-6 fatty acids, and from these your body can make any of the other fats that it needs.

Essential Fatty Acids
Those fats that must be consumed as part of the diet because they are necessary for normal metabolism and cannot be made in the body from other fats.

They are important in cell membrane function, inflammation, platelet aggregation, immunity, hormone balance, blood vessel function, glucose regulation and insulin sensitivity, and enzyme function.

Omega-3 oils in the diet include alpha-linolenic acid (from seeds, nuts, and vegetables) and EPA and DHA from oily fish. The best vegetarian source is flaxseed. Flaxseeds contain about one-third oil, and 50 percent of that is alpha-linolenic acid (also found in walnuts, but in smaller amounts). Alpha-linolenic acid is converted in the body to EPA and DHA. However, sometimes the conversion is inadequate for the full benefits of this oil, and fish oil supplements become important for therapeutic effects. Omega-6 oil (cis-linoleic acid) comes primarily from seeds, nuts, beans, and whole grains, as well as some vegetables. Polyunsaturated fatty acids help to reduce cholesterol levels and blood pressure.

Supplements of omega-3 oils from fish reduce inflammation and decrease platelet aggregation. Scientific studies show that fish oil in the diet or as supplements can reduce the incidence of sudden cardiac death. It can also reduce the recurrence of heart attacks in those who have already had one. For example, in a study of 122 subjects and 118 controls, all of whom had just had a heart attack, those given EPA (eicosapentaenoic acid from fish oil) had one-third fewer cardiac events, including heart attacks, and 40 percent fewer deaths after one year. (A group given 2.9 grams of mustard oil, which is a rich vegetarian source of omega-3, had almost as good results.)

These subjects also improved in other ways. Those who received the fish oil or mustard oil had significantly fewer cardiac arrhythmias, and they had less abnormal enlargement of their ventricles. In addition, the treatment group had less chest pain (angina pectoris), so they felt better. The treatment consisted of just over 1,000 milligrams of EPA daily, which is equal to about five capsules of a common supplement.

When eating fish as a source of omega-3 fatty acids, it is important to choose those that are not contaminated with heavy metals such as mercury, or industrial toxins, such as PCBs and dioxin. Farmed fish, such as salmon, tend to be higher in toxins than wild fish. Government agencies tend to be protective of industry, so when they tell you it is safe to eat some of the fish with higher levels of toxins, you need to be skeptical. They perform what they call risk-benefit ratios, and if the potential benefits outweigh the risks, they say it is safe. This ignores the fact that you can get the same benefits without the risks by making better dietary choices.

As reported in a number of studies, high doses of

fish oils can reduce blood pressure over a three-month period. The studies are not all consistent, but the doses need to be carefully assessed, because some protocols do not use adequate doses to get the desired effects. Nevertheless, it is likely that fish oil is only one part of a comprehensive approach to treating hypertension, which requires dietary change, exercise, stress management, and a variety of other supplements.

Another fatty acid source is a special omega-6 fatty acid called gamma-linolenic acid, or GLA. GLA is found primarily in evening primrose oil and borage oil, both of which are available as supplements. No food source is particularly high in GLA, although it is made in the body from linoleic acid, if all of the necessary enzymes are functioning well. Unfortunately, this is not always the case, so supplements become very valuable therapeutically. GLA has anti-inflammatory properties, and it also reduces platelet aggregation and relaxes blood vessels to improve blood flow, helping to control blood pressure. Some studies suggest that it also helps to lower cholesterol levels.

The precise dose of essential fatty acids that an individual requires and the balance of the omega-3 and omega-6 series that is needed are not clear. Some products on the market claim to contain the ideal balance, but the variation among individuals with different metabolism, various dietary habits, and different health conditions makes this unlikely. Doses may need to be adjusted depending on individual response, but the typical dose of flaxseed oil is 1 to 3 tablespoons per day. One tablespoon of seeds provides about 1 teaspoon of oil.

Capsules of 1,000 milligrams of fish oil concentrates typically contain 300 milligrams of omega-3 oils (a combination of EPA and DHA). Effective doses of EPA and DHA from fish range from two to ten capsules daily, and higher doses have been used for inflammatory conditions, such as arthritis. The most common dose of GLA is 240 milligrams daily. This amount is found in six capsules of evening primrose oil, or one capsule of borage oil, in which it is more concentrated. Some people benefit from taking higher doses of GLA.

Taurine

Taurine is an amino acid, but it is one that is not incorporated into proteins. It has several functions in the body unrelated to proteins or enzymes. Taurine is part of bile, which helps absorb fats and fat-soluble vitamins through the intestinal lining. It is also important for heart muscle function, neurological activity, and cell membrane function. Taurine is a sulfur-containing amino acid, but is not essential in the diet, as it is made from the amino acid L-cysteine, which also contains sulfur and has its own functions. Without taurine, transport of potassium into cells is impaired, leading to arrhythmias that can be fatal (this happened to some people on an inadequate liquid-protein diet in the early 1980s).

Taurine helps to increase the contraction strength of the heart muscle, similar to the effect of a common medication, digitalis, and as such it can help with heart failure, and be valuable in the management of arrhythmias. In a study of seventeen subjects with heart failure due to coronary disease or cardiomyopathy, treatment with 3,000 milligrams of taurine daily led to improvement in their EKGs and in their ejection fraction within six weeks (in this study the results were better than in those receiving coenzyme Q_{10}, but they were only receiving 30 milligrams of CoQ_{10}).

In another study of congestive heart failure, twenty-four patients were administered 4,000 milligrams of taurine daily, and within four weeks, nineteen of the patients were much improved. Of the fifteen patients who were designated as class III or IV heart failure (class IV being the most severe), thirteen improved to the class II level within eight weeks.

When nineteen young people with borderline hypertension were studied, the ten who were treated for seven days with 6,000 milligrams of taurine saw an average 9-point drop in their systolic blood pressure, and a 4-point drop in their diastolic pressure. At the same time, their adrenal stress hormone was found to be lower with treatment. These improvements are highly significant in protecting people from the chronic effects of increased blood pressure, even if it is not high enough to be considered hypertension.

In animal studies, abnormal heart rhythms, including serious ventricular arrhythmias, can be greatly diminished with taurine treatment. In a study of rats, taurine treatment reduced lethal ventricular fibrillation by more than one-half compared to the untreated group. Typical doses of taurine for heart failure, blood pressure control, or arrhythmias range from 1,000 to 4,000 milligrams twice a day.

Arginine

Arginine is another amino acid that is part of some proteins, but it also has functions that are independent of proteins. It is important for wound healing and for hormone secretion, and it stimulates immune function. Arginine is a precursor to nitric oxide, a substance also known as "endothelial-derived relaxing factor." This is produced by the cells that line the arteries, and causes relaxation of the blood vessel muscle, opening up the channel for blood flow. Because of this effect, arginine can help lower blood pressure and improve circulation to the heart and other organs.

Supplements of arginine that go beyond what is found in food have a number of therapeutic effects. Surgical patients who are given supplements of arginine have one- third to one-half as many infections and get out of the hospital 20 to 25 percent faster. (In most of these studies the patients were also given omega-3 fatty acids from fish oil, so the benefits are not exclusive to the arginine.)

A number of small studies show that arginine supplementation can lower systolic blood pressure by 6 points and diastolic blood pressure by 5 points. In one study, fifteen subjects with congestive heart failure were given 5,500 to 12,000 milligrams of arginine for six weeks and placebo for another six weeks, in random sequence. The arginine led to improved blood flow, greater walking distance, and overall reduction in heart-failure symptoms. In a German study using 8,000 milligrams of arginine, blood vessel dilation was four times greater with the supplement than in those who just continued with regular treatment. (Adding exercise to the program enhances function even more.)

Using arginine supplements to treat patients with intermittent claudication (leg pain on exercise due to atherosclerosis) is also beneficial. In a placebo-controlled trial, forty-one patients were given high doses of arginine. After only two weeks, walking distance before pain began was 66 percent higher than before treatment. The benefits were maintained for ten weeks, at which time the study ended.

Nitric oxide is the substance that is released during sexual arousal in men to open up the penile blood vessels and lead to an erection. Medications for erectile dysfunction release nitric oxide, which works to restore sexual functioning. As the nitric oxide precursor, arginine is thought to work similarly to these medications, if taken shortly before sexual activity. Some studies suggest that it is beneficial to take 4,000 to 5,000 milligrams of arginine to achieve this effect. In one study using 5,000 milligrams, 31 percent of men reported improved sexual function with arginine compared to only 12 percent of men on the placebo.

One caution is that some people might respond to high doses of arginine with a recurrence of herpes virus outbreaks, but this has not been confirmed. Supplements of the amino acid lysine would help balance the arginine and reduce the risk of viral recurrence. Typical doses of arginine range from 2,000 milligrams to 6,000 milligrams daily. Higher doses might be effective for some situations.

Policosanol

Policosanol is a mixture of waxy alcohols derived from sugar cane, rice bran oil, or wheat germ oil. Approximately seven of these waxy substances are common in the product called Policosanol, but one of the most prominent is one called octacosanol and, in the past, this name has been used to refer to the product. One effect of Policosanol is to lower serum cholesterol, but it also has more profound effects that provide benefits far beyond its cholesterol effect.

In addition to lowering total cholesterol, Policosanol lowers the LDL cholesterol, raises the good HDL cholesterol, and decreases the serum triglyceride level. In recent years doctors have been recommending a class of drugs called "statins" to lower cholesterol, often even for people with normal serum levels, noting that these drugs have other benefits in stabilizing atherosclerotic plaque (rupture of unstable plaque can lead to heart attacks), protecting endothelial cells, and possibly having anti-inflammatory properties. When faced with alternatives to these drugs for treating cholesterol, doctors often point out all of these other benefits of the drugs. However, in looking at the research on Policosanol, it is clear that it has many of the same benefits as statin drugs, but without the potential side effects.

Policosanol is better than statins on many counts. In a comparative study with pravastatin, Policosanol offered greater protection of the endothelium, better inhibition of platelet aggregation, and improved HDL levels. In animal studies, when compared to lovastatin, Policosanol is better at reducing arterial thickening.

While the most effective statin, Lipitor, is slightly better at lowering total cholesterol than Policosanol, it does not raise HDL as Policsanol does, so the heart disease risk reduction provided by the two substances is identical. Policosanol is equal to Lipitor at lowering triglyceride levels, and it protects LDL cholesterol from oxidation. Oxidized LDL is a risk factor for atherosclerosis.

Policosanol has further clinical benefits. In a study of intermittent claudication (pain in the legs on exercise), Policosanol treatment increased walking distance by 60 percent within six months, and at the end of two years by 200 to 300 percent. A recent five-month study showed that Policosanol was better than lovastatin for improving claudication, and that it also lowered serum fibrinogen, a blood-clotting protein that is a risk factor for heart disease.

Statins can cause a severe muscle breakdown called rhabdomyolysis, with leakage of muscle-cell contents into the circulation. This is a serious condition, and one of the statins was removed from the market because of this side effect. In addition, statin drugs all reduce the production of coenzyme Q_{10}, increasing the risk and severity of congestive heart failure. Comprehensive reviews show that while statins may reduce the incidence of heart disease, and reduce cardiac deaths, they may not reduce overall mortality.

The statin drugs are among the more expensive medical treatments for heart disease, with potentially serious side effects. The evidence shows that patients should be given Policosanol, which is far less expensive and equally or even more effective. If you do decide to take the statins, it is important to also take coenzyme Q_{10} at the same time to avoid a deficiency of this important substance.

Some of the Policosanol brands on the market are not the same as the sugarcane derivative on which most of the research has been done. Their profile of waxy alcohols is different, and may not be as effective. The product derived from sugar cane is the one to look for, although future research may well prove that some other sources are valuable. The typical dose of Policosanol is 20 milligrams per day. Benefits are seen with as little as 10 milligrams, but the effect is greater with the larger dose. It appears that doses higher than 20 milligrams offer little extra benefit.

Red Yeast Rice

Red yeast is a fermentation product grown on rice that contains substances called monacolins, and may have other active components as well. Supplements of red yeast rice lower serum cholesterol levels. The effect is likely caused by the inhibition of a liver enzyme that is essential in the metabolic pathway of cholesterol production, called HMG CoA reductase. This is the same enzyme that is inhibited by statin drugs, and one of the monacolins, called monacolin K, is identical to the drug lovastatin, but it is present in much lower amounts in the red yeast rice.

The Food and Drug Administration has blocked the sale of Cholestin, a standardized extract of this natural product, due to a patent-infringement lawsuit by the drug company making lovastatin. As natural products cannot be patented, it is unclear how this could happen, other than as a result of the financial power of the drug companies. As the FDA had already granted a patent to the related drugs, availability of the natural product would have inhibited sale of the drug when it was found to have similar effects.

The amount of the active component of red yeast rice is small in nonstandardized products, but it is still effective. In a Chinese study of sixty heart patients, one-half were given 1,200 milligrams of a red yeast rice extract and half a placebo. After six weeks, the patients on the red yeast rice had significant lowering of their fasting triglyceride levels, as well as lipoprotein (a), and they had the additional benefit of reduction of their CRP level (the inflammatory marker that is a risk factor for heart disease).

A similar study of fifty heart patients by the same researchers showed that the same dose of red yeast rice led to a 20 percent decline in total cholesterol, a 34 percent decline in LDL cholesterol, a 32 percent decline in triglyceride levels, and an 18 percent increase in serum HDL. These are highly significant improvements in heart disease risk factors.

Because the active component of red yeast rice has the same effect as lovastatin, it would be wise to take coenzyme Q_{10} along with this supplement. Typical doses of the red yeast rice are from 500 to 1,000 milligrams, two or three times a day.

D-Ribose

D-ribose is a five-carbon sugar that is part of DNA (deoxyribonucleic acid) and RNA (ribonucleic acid), and it is essential for energy storage as part of the energy storage molecule, ATP. In times of stress on the heart, D-ribose can provide extra energy for the heart muscle, leading to increased exercise tolerance in heart patients before they develop angina.

After an episode of low oxygen to the heart, the production of ATP is limited and takes up to seventy-two hours to be restored. Supplements of D-ribose can enhance the ATP production so that energy is restored to the heart muscle sooner. Large doses may be necessary to achieve this effect. In one study, patients with severe coronary disease had treadmill testing for two days, and then were given either 60 grams of D-ribose or a placebo daily for three days. On day five, they had a repeat treadmill test. The supplemented group did significantly better than the placebo group in exercise duration before symptoms developed.

Supplements of D-ribose also help patients with congestive heart failure, as it again improves the functional capacity of the heart muscle. In fifteen patients with coronary disease and congestive heart failure, supplements of D-ribose for three weeks improved quality of life and stress-test function, and enhanced the contraction ability of the heart. Because of these properties of D-ribose, it is also likely to help with arrhythmias.

Although high doses of D-ribose are quite safe, it is also likely that even smaller doses over time would be beneficial for the heart muscle in patients with angina or other signs of coronary disease. A typical dose for heart patients is 5 grams of D-ribose three times a day, but higher or lower doses are also beneficial.

CHAPTER 6

HERBAL SUPPLEMENTS FOR THE HEART

Substances derived from plants have been a staple of medical therapy through the ages. In fact, many modern drugs are derivatives or synthetic modifications of plant products. Botanical medicine is often less expensive and safer than conventional drugs (but not always). Whether or not botanical products are technically herbal products depends on which part of the plant they come from, but they are commonly lumped together under the term "herbs."

Herbal therapies are enjoying a surge in popularity with the interest in natural medicine, the desire for less toxic therapies, and the need for less expensive treatments. The medical profession and researchers are increasingly studying and using these therapies in practice and in laboratories, and the amount of research on herbal medicine has added further support to their value.

Standardized Herbs

Although herbs have a long history of use for medicinal purposes, it is only relatively recently that they have been analyzed to reveal their most active components. These active chemicals are commonly present in very variable amounts in herbs, depending on where and how they are grown, soil quality, when they are harvested, the amount of rain and sun, and other factors. Standardized herbs have guaranteed specific amounts of the known, active herbal components, as well as the other factors that might be of help but are not as well studied.

The German government formed a Commission

(Commission E) to conduct a review of the clinical value of many herbs in common therapeutic use. In order to control as many variables as possible, the main focus of their review was on standardized herbs. Commission E has published the results of their review in a monograph, concluding that many herbs do have the effects that are claimed for them, as long as they have the active components. In order to benefit the most from herbal treatments, I recommend that you choose standardized herbs.

Curcumin

Curcumin is a standardized extract of turmeric, the intense yellow-orange spice found in curry powder. It is standardized to 90 to 95 percent curcumin. Curcumin is actually a mixture of several antioxidant flavonoids collectively called curcuminoids. As an antioxidant, free-radical scavenger, curcumin supplements can reduce the level of damaging "lipid peroxides" in the blood, and at the same time lower total cholesterol, and raise the good HDL levels by as much as 39 percent in one study. Another study showed that the decrease in cholesterol is due to increased lipid metabolism, rather than inhibition of production, so the mechanism is quite different from that of red yeast rice or statin drugs.

In an animal study, diabetic rats were treated with curcumin and it helped to lower blood sugar and reduce some of the other changes of sugar metabolism that are associated with the long-term complications of diabetes. Curcumin also enhanced the activity of an antioxidant enzyme called glutathione peroxidase. Improving insulin sensitivity and increasing oxidation protection are two important mechanisms for protection against cardiovascular disease.

Curcumin also inhibits platelet aggregation, reducing the likelihood of clotting within blood vessels. It also has anti-inflammatory properties, and as a result it can lower the cardiovascular risks associated with inflammation and elevated CRP levels. In animal studies, curcumin lowered inflammatory markers as much as ibuprofen (Advil). Aspirin is often recommended for heart patients to reduce platelet aggregation and inflammatory markers, but it appears that you can get the same benefits from curcumin (and many other supplements) without the risks of taking drugs. (Even low-dose aspirin has risks to the kidneys, brain, and gastrointestinal tract.)

A number of animal studies show that curcumin protects the heart from a variety of damage sources. In addition it has the side benefit of protecting against a number of cancers, and it is likely to protect the brain against Alzheimer's disease. The usual dose of curcumin is 300 to 500 milligrams, taken two or three times a day as an anti-inflammatory. A small amount taken daily may offer protection against brain aging and heart disease. For people who already have atherosclerotic heart disease it is likely to be beneficial to take it regularly.

Garlic

The culinary use of garlic is ancient, and it also has a long history of therapeutic use in traditional medicine. In fact, garlic has so many documented therapeutic uses that it creates skepticism in the minds of many doctors. Garlic contains many sulfur compounds, including allicin and ajoene, and garlic supplements have relatives of these substances in varying amounts, depending on processing, but there is no standardization for garlic products. Garlic appears to lower blood pressure and cholesterol in some but not all studies. It also inhibits platelet aggregation, aids in the breakdown of blood clots, and inhibits the production of some inflammatory substances.

Garlic appears to increase the production of nitric oxide in the body by increasing the activity of the enzyme required for its synthesis. Increased nitric oxide enhances blood flow by relaxing blood vessels, and lowers blood pressure. In a controlled Russian study, eighty-five subjects taking one preparation of garlic at 600 milligrams daily had a significant lowering of both systolic and diastolic blood pressure.

In a study of 100 pregnant women, garlic supplements significantly lowered blood pressure and total cholesterol levels. A German study of forty-seven patients with moderate hypertension found that after twelve weeks, diastolic blood pressure was reduced from 102 to 89 with garlic supplements. In the treatment group cholesterol and triglycerides were also lowered with treatment. No changes occurred in the placebo group in either blood pressure or lipid levels. In a controlled study of 152 subjects, garlic led to a reduction of plaque in the carotid and femoral arteries over a four-year period.

Most garlic preparations available as supplements are deodorized, making them more acceptable for daily consumption. (Capsules sold as "odorless" garlic oil are not really deodorized, and they are not as concentrated as the deodorized or aged products.) Many manufacturers make claims that theirs is the only effective product, or the best one available. However, most of the preparations available from reliable companies are effective if taken in the therapeutic dose ranges, and no specific preparation stands out as the best. Typical daily doses are from 500 to 1,000 milligrams of deodorized garlic, two to three times a day.

Ginkgo Biloba

Ginkgo biloba is an ancient tree. Substances derived from it have a long history of use in traditional medical therapy. Ginkgo leaf extracts contain flavonoid-like compounds with antioxidant activity, and lactones that are protective of small blood vessels and nerves. These substances improve circulation in the brain and eyes. Studies show that ginkgo supplements can slow the progression of Alzheimer's disease.

Animal studies show that ginkgo extracts can lower blood pressure, improve nitric oxide activity, reduce thrombosis, and have antioxidant effects. In patients with intermittent claudication, ginkgo can improve walking distance before the onset of pain in the legs. In a study of 111 patients with athero-sclerosis in the legs, a daily dose of 120 milligrams of ginkgo extract for twenty-four weeks led to a nearly 50 percent improvement in pain-free walking distance.

Some research suggests that one mechanism of action of ginkgo is to lower the blood levels of stress hormones, leading to reduced blood pressure and less spasm of arteries. Standardized ginkgo extracts contain 24 percent flavone glycosides, and 6 percent lactones. For people taking aspirin to inhibit platelets, ginkgo might well be a good substitute (along with many other dietary supplements with similar effects), and they should be cautious about taking both together. The typical dose of ginkgo is 120 milligrams daily. Some people may benefit from higher doses.

Hawthorn

Hawthorn is a hedge or small tree with red berries. The leaves and flowers of hawthorn (and to some extent the berries) contain antioxidant flavonoids and anthocyanins that have therapeutic properties for heart function, and they also inhibit the produc-tion of inflammatory substances. Hawthorn extract relaxes blood vessels to improve blood flow and it can improve the function of the heart muscle. It is an effective inhibitor of the oxidation of LDL choles-terol, with the potential to reduce damage to the arteries.

In animal studies, the extract can reduce arrhyth-mias and lower blood pressure. Human research is also positive. A study of thirty patients with mild con-gestive heart failure showed that hawthorn supple-ments lowered blood pressure a small amount after eight weeks and improved performance on a sta-tionary bicycle, including less shortness of breath; it also led to a reduction of subjective health complaints. Another eight-week placebo-controlled study of 143 patients showed that hawthorn supplements improved exercise tolerance and reduced shortness of breath and fatigue.

In a twenty-four-week study of over 1,000 patients with heart failure, hawthorn led to an 83 percent reduction of ankle swelling and frequency of nighttime urination. Exercise tolerance was also improved in the treatment group, and the ejection fraction (a measure of heart muscle function) was better after treatment. Two-thirds of the patients reported feeling better with the hawthorn treatment, and physician evaluation showed a good or very good response. Hawthorn has also been suggested to help with angina.

Typical doses of hawthorn range from 250 to 500 milligrams of standardized extract, taken twice a day. The standardized extract contains 2.2 percent of the bioflavonoid vitexin.

CHAPTER 7

A COMPREHENSIVE HEART-TREATMENT PROGRAM

Preventing and treating heart and vascular diseases involves a healthy lifestyle, exercise, diet, and stress reduction, as well as a variety of dietary supplements. A recommendation for dietary supplements to assist you does not mean that you can abandon the other important healthy choices. Most heart and vascular diseases are related to oxidation, toxicity, and inflammation, and they may be brought on by obesity, environmental exposures, inappropriate fats or too much fat in the diet, smoking, and other lifestyle choices.

Supplement treatments for the common heart conditions are similar to each other, but with some differences for each problem. Common recommendations are not meant as medical advice or as a substitute for a proper evaluation and treatment by a physician, but it is a good idea to find a physician who is familiar with nutrition and dietary supplements, including herbs.

How to Begin

When creating a supplement program, I recommend starting with a comprehensive, high-potency multivitamin/mineral combination. This will simplify your program and reduce the number of different supplements you might need. Most of these combinations require four to six pills a day, depending on the brand, size of pill, and potency. The one I most commonly recommend contains potent amounts of the B complex vitamins, vitamins C and E, and calcium and magnesium in equal amounts, as well as all of the other basic nutrients. I will refer to this as the "Basic Multiple," and it has the following formula contained in a daily dose of six tablets:

Vitamin A	5,000 IU
Vitamin C	1,200 mg
Beta-carotene (natural)	15,000 IU
Vitamin D_3	400 IU
Vitamin E (natural)	400 IU
Thiamine (B_1)	100 mg
Riboflavin (B_2)	50 mg
Niacinamide (B_3)	150 mg
Niacin (B_3)	40 mg
Pyridoxine (B_6)	100 mg
Folate (folic acid)	800 mcg
Vitamin B_{12}	250 mcg
Biotin	300 mcg
Pantothenic acid	250 mg
Calcium (citrate/ascorbate)	500 mg
Magnesium (aspartate/ascorbate)	500 mg
Iodine	200 mcg
Zinc	30 mg
Selenium	200 mcg
Chromium	200 mcg
Copper	3 mg
Manganese	20 mg
Molybdenum	100 mcg
Citrus bioflavonoids	100 mg
PABA	50 mg
Vanadium	50 mcg
Boron	3 mg

You can check with health food stores and mail order vitamins for comparable formulas. You might find others that are similar but not exactly the same. You can make up the specific differences by adding a missing nutrient separately. Note that this formula does not include iron. Excess iron is associated with an increased risk of heart disease, and I do not recommend it unless you have a specific need based on a medical evaluation.

I almost always recommend taking supplements after breakfast and supper, partly because they seem to work better with food, and they are easier on the stomach. In addition, people often neglect to take supplements in the middle of the day, or if they have to remember to take them without food. While it may be true that some supplements, such as amino acids, may work better separate from meals, they won't work at all if you forget to take them.

Managing Specific Problems

In addition to improving general well-being and preventing disease, dietary supplements are valuable aids in modifying risk factors and treating specific disorders. Of course, you don't need to wait until you have a specific problem, but if you have known risk factors or disease, dietary supplements can help.

High Cholesterol

Cholesterol elevation in the serum is a risk factor for heart disease, although it is clearly not the only factor. Nevertheless, people with cholesterol levels below 150 milligrams/deciliter, do not get atherosclerotic heart disease, and it is not harmful to have cholesterol in that range. The most important first step in controlling cholesterol is to eat a healthy diet (as I will discuss later) and exercise. A number of supplements lower cholesterol but you do not need to take all of them in order to benefit. I suggest taking the basic supplements and then choosing a few from the others in the following list to see what works for you, and changing to others or different doses if you do not see the desired results.

SUPPLEMENTS	AM	PM
Basic Multiple Formula	3	3
L-Carnitine, 500 mg	2	2
Chromium, 200 mcg	1	1
Coenzyme Q_{10}, 200 mg	1	
Fish oil, 1,000 mg (with 300 mg of EPA/DHA)	2	2
Garlic, deodorized or aged, 500 mg	1–2	1–2
Niacin (inositol hexaniacinate), 400–500 mg	2–3	2–3
Policosanol, 10 mg	1	1
Red Yeast Rice, 500 mg	2	1
Vitamin C, 1,000 mg	2	2
Vitamin E, 400 IU natural, mixed		1

High Homocysteine Levels

High homocysteine is best managed by taking supplements. The following program includes the basic nutrients for overall heart health plus some specifics that help to lower the serum homocysteine level.

SUPPLEMENTS	AM	PM
Basic Multiple Formula	3	3
Cobalamin (vitamin B_{12}), 1,000–2,500 mcg	1	1
Folic acid (folate), 5,000 mcg	1	
Pyridoxine (vitamin B_6), 100 mg	1	
Vitamin C, 1,000 mg	2	2
Vitamin E, 400 IU natural, mixed		1

High CRP

Chronic inflammation is a risk factor for heart disease, regardless of the cause, and elevated CRP is one marker of inflammation. Many dietary supplements have anti-inflammatory properties. I include them in the program for people with high serum levels of CRP, in addition to other protective supplements.

SUPPLEMENTS	AM	PM
Basic Multiple Formula	3	3
Curcumin, 300 mg	1–2	1–2
Fish oil, 1,000 mg (with 300 mg of EPA/DHA)	2–3	2–3
Niacin (inositol hexaniacinate), 400–500 mg	2	2
Vitamin C, 1,000 mg	2	2
Vitamin E, 400 IU natural, mixed		1

Arteriosclerotic Heart Disease (including Angina)

For prevention, I recommend the Basic Multiple, as well as an additional 2,000 milligrams of vitamin C, and as risk increases with age or family history of heart disease, or having smoked tobacco, I would add an extra 400 IU of vitamin E, as well as 100 milligrams of coenzyme Q$_{10}$.

For treatment of someone with symptoms, I would suggest increasing supplements according to the following program (in alphabetical order—not in order of importance), with amounts partly dependent on the severity of the disease, and not necessarily taking all of them in the early stages of heart disease:

SUPPLEMENTS	AM	PM
Basic Multiple Formula	3	3
Arginine, 500 mg	2–4	2–4
Coenzyme Q$_{10}$, 200 mg	1	
Fish oil, 1,000 mg (with 300 mg of EPA/DHA)	2	2
Ginkgo biloba extract, 60 mg	1	1
Hawthorn, standardized, 250 mg	1	1
L-Carnitine, 500 mg	2	2
Magnesium aspartate, 200 mg	1	1
Policosanol, 10 mg	1	1
Vitamin C, 1,000 mg	2	2
Vitamin E, 400 IU natural, mixed		1
D-Ribose, 5–10 g	1–2	1–2

Congestive Heart Failure

Treatment of congestive heart failure involves a number of supplements, the most important of which may well be coenzyme Q_{10}. In many ways, the program is similar to the treatment of atherosclerosis, and that is often the underlying cause of heart failure. Heart failure is a serious condition, and requires medical management. The supplement program that I recommend is comprehensive because of the nature of the condition. The following supplement list leaves room for modification depending on the heart failure classification, with the higher doses for more severe conditions:

SUPPLEMENTS	AM	PM
Basic Multiple Formula	3	3
Coenzyme Q_{10}, 200 mg (chewable tablets)	1–2	
Fish oil, 1,000 mg (with 300 mg of EPA/DHA)	2	2
Hawthorn, standardized, 250 mg	1	1
L-Carnitine, 500 mg	2–3	2–3
Magnesium (aspartate), 200 mg	1	1–2
Taurine, 500 mg	2–4	2–4
Vitamin C, 1,000 mg	2	2
Vitamin E, 400 IU natural, mixed		1
D-Ribose, 5 g	1–2	1–2

Hypertension

High blood pressure adds significantly to the risk of heart disease and atherosclerosis in other parts of the body, including the brain, the legs, and the kidneys. Controlling blood pressure is a model for a comprehensive approach to managing health problems, because it is influenced by diet, exercise, stress management, and dietary supplements. A program for blood pressure includes the following supplements, but you may find that a few are all you need. For higher blood pressures or if you are not following the rest of your health program, you may need higher doses of some supplements.

SUPPLEMENTS	AM	PM
Basic Multiple Formula	3	3
Arginine, 500 mg	2–3	2–3
Coenzyme Q$_{10}$, 200 mg (chewable tablets)	1	
Fish oil, 1,000 mg (with 300 mg of EPA/DHA)	2	2
Garlic, deodorized, 500 mg	1–2	1–2
Hawthorn, 250 mg	1	1
Magnesium aspartate, 200 mg		1
Vitamin C, 1,000 mg	2	2
Vitamin E, 400 IU natural, mixed		1

Arrhythmias

Abnormal heart rhythms have a variety of causes, and a full medical evaluation is important to understanding what is underlying the condition. It may be relatively benign, and it may be a sign of something more serious. The following supplements may help in a variety of arrhythmias, whether or not you need any medication in addition. Depending on the cause of the arrhythmia, other supplements may also help the treatment or to prevent some of the complications of the abnormal rhythm.

SUPPLEMENTS	AM	PM
Basic Multiple Formula	3	3
Fish oil, 1,000 mg (with 300 mg of EPA/DHA)	2	2
Hawthorn, 250 mg	1	1
Magnesium aspartate, 200 mg	1	1
Taurine, 5,000 mg	3	3
Vitamin C, 1,000 mg	2	2
Vitamin E, 400 IU natural, mixed		1
D-Ribose, 5 g	1	1

CHAPTER 8

OTHER TREATMENTS FOR THE HEART

Although nutrition, exercise, stress management, and dietary supplements are powerful prevention and treatment methods, sometimes it is necessary to have more vigorous intervention. This may include medication and surgery, but other treatments are also available that may help you avoid the need for these therapies. One such treatment that I highly recommend for heart patients is intravenous chelation therapy.

Chelation Therapy for Circulation

For treating heart disease, chelation therapy is the intravenous administration of a synthetic amino acid called ethylene diamine tetraacetic acid, or EDTA. The treatment takes about three hours, and is usually administered two to three times a week in a doctor's office. The use of chelation therapy in medicine was originally developed for its benefits in ridding the body of toxic heavy metals, such as lead, cadmium, and arsenic, as the EDTA binds with these metals and carries them out in the urine. The early researchers noticed that their patients who also happened to have heart disease were reporting that their angina was getting better with the treatment. EDTA also removes excess iron, which has been associated with an increased risk of heart disease.

Chelation Therapy
For heart disease, refers to the intravenous administration of a synthetic amino acid (EDTA) to remove toxic metals and enhance magnesium levels in cells to improve heart function.

Numerous studies from the 1950s through the 1980s showed the many benefits of chelation for heart disease and its complications, as well as for atherosclerosis in the legs (intermittent claudication), and cerebrovascular disease (strokes and brain degeneration). It has also been shown to be a very safe treatment when administered according to current protocols. However, EDTA chelation became quite controversial in the 1970s when coronary artery bypass surgery became a more popular treatment within the medical community. Still, a few thousand doctors practice chelation therapy, and the evidence in its favor has prompted the National Institutes of Health Center for Complementary and Alternative Medicine to finance a 3-million-dollar study of the treatment.

Oral treatment with EDTA has been promoted by some doctors as being valuable as an alternative to intravenous chelation treatment. However, oral chelation with EDTA has not been demonstrated to help heart disease, and EDTA taken orally is not well absorbed. In addition, regular consumption of large doses of EDTA has never been studied for safety in the same way as intravenous therapy. For heart disease, oral EDTA therapy is not a substitute for intravenous treatment.

Most doctors who do chelation therapy belong to the American College for Advancement in Medicine (ACAM), and they can be located by contacting the organization. ACAM conducts training programs for doctors in nutrition, preventive medicine, anti-aging medicine, and other treatments, as well as chelation therapy. Chelation therapy is only one part of a comprehensive treatment for heart disease. It does not interfere with other treatments, and doing chelation does not mean that you cannot also have medical or surgical treatments.

Oral chelating substances do have value in treating disease, possibly including heart disease, but these are different from EDTA. For example, dimercaptosuccinic acid (DMSA) is quite effective in removing mercury from tissues, and taken orally in small amounts it is quite safe. High tissue levels of mercury have been associated with an increased risk of heart disease, so removing mercury is valuable.

Mercury is toxic in many other ways. It binds with selenium, preventing this nutrient from working as an antioxidant cofactor. It also binds with sulfur-containing antioxidant enzymes, leading to more free-radical damage. Mercury may induce the oxidation of LDL cholesterol. In addition, it increases blood clotting and platelet aggregation, induces inflammation, and damages endothelial cells. EDTA is not very effective at removing mercury, so it may be necessary to do more than one form of chelation treatment for all of the potential benefits.

CHAPTER 9

DIET AND LIFESTYLE TO PROTECT THE HEART

Diet and lifestyle play very important roles in preventing and treating heart disease. It is important to have specific information about how to implement healthy changes in your life in order to achieve the greatest benefit. These healthy practices are also likely to make you feel better and prevent or even treat problems that you may already have. Any change that you make will be helpful, so it is not a failure if you are unable to do it all, but the more you do the more you will benefit.

Dietary Guidelines

Dietary information available to the public is sometimes confusing and often inaccurate. While many fads come and go in an effort to sell books to manage obesity, the science behind healthy dietary guidelines is fairly consistent and very clear. The healthiest diet is high in vegetables, fruits, seeds, nuts, whole grains, and legumes (including soybean products), with some fish (wild and uncontaminated, such as wild salmon and water-packed sardines). It is also low in meats, dairy products, saturated fats, hydrogenated oils, refined foods, and heavily processed foods.

Such a diet is the most likely diet to prevent and reverse heart disease and mortality from all causes. This diet is also lowest in environmental toxins, including pesticides, toxic metals, and industrial waste products, although it is always best to select organic products (whether you choose to include meats or not) to further reduce these poisons.

This healthy diet is high in fiber, essential vitamins

and minerals, flavonoids, antioxidants, and other health-enhancing phytochemicals. In addition, it is adequate (but not high) in protein and low in fat, but it provides the essential fatty acids that are so important for heart health. If you want to add eggs to this diet, choose those that are produced with organic farming methods. They are generally high in omega-3 fatty acids, and they are not exposed to hormones and growth stimulants. If you add dairy products, choose organic, low-fat or nonfat varieties. The best dairy product is probably yogurt, but be sure to avoid the flavored ones that are high in sugar.

Meats from land animals, including poultry, and dairy products are unnecessary in the diet, although very small amounts are not likely to do too much harm. Animal products accumulate more toxins than plants, and animals are treated with antibiotics and estrogenic hormones to increase growth and reproduction. They are often given genetically engineered growth hormone (BST, or rBGH), to fatten them up and speed them to market (even farmed salmon may be given growth hormone). Residues of some of the hormones and antibiotics stay in the flesh, leading to a rash of new problems with antibiotic-resistant bacteria and hormone irregularities. With the recent scares about mad cow disease (bovine spongiform encephalopathy, or BSE) it increasingly appears that avoiding meat is a healthy dietary decision. However, the association of meat consumption with heart disease is a much more serious risk.

In order to be healthy, you need to avoid sources of refined sugars (such as candies and ice cream), as well as artificial sweeteners. Also avoid white flour or refined flour products (pastries, white breads, cakes, pies, and any foods of a related nature), white rice, and other highly processed foods. Avoid artificial flavors, colors and preservatives, and keep caffeine beverages to a minimum. Particularly try to eliminate sodas and chocolate drinks, as well as doughnuts and other deep fried foods.

There is significant evidence that consuming some alcohol, such as wine and beer, is helpful to prevent heart attacks, although other beverages and foods, such as grape juice, may provide similar benefits. If you have hypertension, it is probably best to avoid alcohol, and if you are not drinking alcohol now, the evidence is not sufficient to suggest that you start just for the potential health benefits. If you do drink, it is best to do so in moderation, but no one can tell you exactly what that is. More than one drink a day is probably not a good idea.

It is most important to avoid all margarine and partially hydrogenated vegetable oils. Polyunsaturated oils have fragile bonds that are subject to oxidation, and the food industry has attempted to stabilize these bonds by adding hydrogen to them so they do not become rancid as readily. Unfortunately, in the process they created fats that do not occur in the diet. These altered fats are called "trans fatty acids," and they are harmful in many ways. Trans fats interfere with normal fat metabolism, they alter the character of cell membranes that contain fat (so that transport of nutrients and waste across those membranes is affected), and they are related to a higher risk of cancer and heart disease. Many processed foods contain these fats, also referred to as vegetable shortening.

It is essential to read labels on all products until you are familiar with the ingredients. The order of ingredients determines the amount of that substance in the product. (First on the list is the highest amount, and last is the lowest.) You will see the amount of fat, saturated fat, protein, sugar, fiber, and sodium on the labels now. Food labels are being changed to include the amount of trans fats that products contain.

If you are trying to eat whole, unprocessed, organic foods, the safest and most reliable grocery store is a health food store. However, even these stores carry products that are not entirely healthy, and might contain refined flour and sugar, among other deleterious substances. Therefore, reading labels is important no matter where you shop.

Try to avoid large amounts of added salt in your food. Tamari (soy sauce) is an alternative to table salt, but this also contains a large amount of salt. If you choose to use it to season your foods, dilute it and use it sparingly. Do not use soy sauce if you require a no-salt diet. Use other herbs and spices including onions and garlic. Try lemon or vinegar for accent to brighten up your food and reduce your intake of salt. You can also replace salt with mixtures of herbs to add zest to your meals, and many herbs have other healthful properties.

For beverages drink water or sparkling spring water; unsweetened fruit juices, diluted with at least an equal amount of filtered or spring water to reduce the sugar concentration; herbal teas; vegetable juice; and grain/cereal coffee-substitutes (Cafix, Postum). If you like coffee, try some water-processed decaffeinated coffee. Buy organic decaf to avoid pesticide residues. Soy milk or plain "Rice Dream" beverages are good on cereals as milk substitutes.

Make fresh salad dressings with herbs, spices, lemon juice or oil and vinegar. Use only extra virgin olive oil, unrefined flaxseed oil or "high oleic" oils that have higher levels of the monounsaturated oils. Do not use dressings with added sweeteners. Many dressings are available with no salt added. These products can usually be found in health food stores, although conventional stores are increasingly carrying healthier products. Avoid those that contain artificial ingredients and hydrogenated oils. Unsweetened catsup and tofu-mayonnaise, with no additives, are also available in health food stores.

While not everyone has the same nutritional requirements, in general, dietary needs are very similar. In order to come up with the right diet for yourself, you need to do some experimentation, but these guidelines should set you on the right path.

The ultimate goal is to maintain a lifetime of health-ful and wholesome eating habits. It is not a quick weight-loss plan, nor is it some fad that is based on marketing or inaccurate interpretation of the sci-ence. This still leaves a wide range of healthy, nutri-tious, and delicious foods from which to choose. Base your choices on a variety of fresh, organic veg-etables, fruits, beans, and whole grains, and add a small amount of fish, and if you choose, organic eggs, and organic, nonfat dairy products.

Dietary Fads

Many dietary fads are based on low carbohydrate plans, and are high in protein and fat. They often ignore the difference between simple carbohydrates, such as sugar and white flour, and complex carbohy-drates, found in whole grains, beans, potatoes, and squashes. The programs I am referring to include the Atkins diet, the "zone" diet, the "blood type" diet, and others.

The medical literature is full of articles on which approaches to diet lead to the healthiest results. Most popularly promoted dietary fads focus simply on weight loss; however, health is not simply weight control, but protection from everyday health prob-lems and prevention and treatment of chronic, debil-itating and lethal diseases, including heart disease. (Of course, it is good if the diet that reduces your risk of heart disease, and also reverses it, at the same time protects you from strokes, hypertension, cancer, diabetes, gout, and osteoporosis, as well as overall mortality.)

Weight Loss Does Not Equal Health

Unlike the medical literature, the popular press is full of a variety of books and articles on diets that sound scientific, but for the most part ignore the most important information—what is the long-term health consequence of their recommendations? These authors propose to help people with weight loss, and their plans might do this, but that is one of their dangers: they lull people into thinking that because they lose weight they are becoming healthier. These diet plans are almost always based on some metabolic gimmick that is supposedly hidden in the medical literature.

They may provide temporary weight loss (no such system has been shown to help people maintain lower weight in the long term—that is, more than a year), but at the expense of long-term health, and the risk of increasing the illnesses mentioned above.

The "Zone" Diet, or the "Danger Zone"

The zone diet proponent, Barry Sears, suggests that the "American experiment with low fat diets has failed," but he is wrong. Americans have not been on a low-fat diet. When he started saying this, Americans had dropped from an extremely high-fat diet (over 40 percent of calories), down to a still very-high intake of 33 percent.

The drop in percent was not from reduced fat, but the result of increased calories from sugar and white flour. The total fat in the diet had not decreased. I agree with Sears that processed and hydrogenated oils have replaced important essential fatty acids from the diet, and that extra refined carbohydrate, and artificial ingredients have increased illness, but the solution is not to eat a diet that is unhealthy for other reasons.

Dr. Sears speaks often about insulin resistance as the cause of obesity. This is a serious metabolic problem that is the result of obesity and lack of exercise. The best treatment for insulin resistance is exercise, reduced caloric intake, and a high fiber diet. Fiber is virtually absent in all animal foods. A number of studies show that high-fiber whole grains actually reduce insulin resistance and are associated with reduced risks of heart disease and diabetes. On the other hand, refined grains increase the risks.

High-protein diets may increase the loss of calcium

in the urine, and possibly lead to an increased risk of osteoporosis. Calcium loss is also increased by phosphorus, which is abundant in animal products. The nitrogen in high-protein diets is a burden on the kidneys and liver. Animal products also increase the risk of gallstones and gout.

The Atkins Diet

This is a high-protein, high-fat diet, with carbohydrates of any sort being considered villainous. No credible scientific evidence shows that people who stay on this diet are healthier, or even that they maintain consistent weight loss, although any of these diets can help people lose weight in the short term, mainly from calorie restriction.

It is hard to imagine a diet being promoted as healthy in which the recommended breakfast consists of eggs, bacon, sausages, cheese and similar foods. If nothing else, such a diet is high in pesticides, antibiotics, and hormones, in addition to the fat and saturated-fat content, which have consistently been associated with increased disease risk. The proponents of the Atkins diet say "well, of course, you should choose organic foods whenever possible." However, I have observed many proponents of these diets, and if what they choose when they are at conferences is any reflection, they eat high animal protein no matter what the source, and they are discounting too much medical science.

Another problem with such diets is the lack of the important phytochemicals found in a wide variety of fruits, vegetables, whole grains, and beans. These are important antioxidants, isoflavones, bioflavonoids, and other protective substances. They are simply not present in animal foods. For example, blueberries were recently shown to be the food with the highest antioxidant levels.

The Blood-Type Diet Craze

In the blood-type diet, author and naturopath Peter

D'Adamo suggests that most people are not adapted genetically to be vegetarian, and that what you need is based on whether your blood type is A, B, AB, or O. Again, no credible scientific data supports this, as no studies have been done on people who choose diets based on their blood type. In fact, people who choose vegetarian diets usually do so for other reasons. If they were ill-adapted to this choice, you would expect more illness among those who were vegetarian for the "wrong" reasons.

But the science shows that people who choose vegetarian diets are healthier. A simple search of the medical literature, which anyone can do easily at the National Library of Medicine website (www. ncbi.nlm.nih.gov/PubMed/), shows that vegetarians have lower rates of heart disease, reduced incidence of many cancers, and less diabetes and hypertension (when you go to the website, just plug in the word "vegetarian" for your search). This information comes from a variety of population groups, epidemiological studies, and intervention studies, and it is consistent, independent of the country in which the research is done. Choosing to eat in a way contrary to the science based on blood type or any other fad is creating an unnecessary health risk.

Relaxation and the Heart

It is now accepted that emotional and psychological stress can contribute to heart disease. Anxiety, depression, and social isolation can make heart failure worse and lead to more hospitalization. Hostility is associated with an increase in coronary heart disease. Just the perception of being under high stress is an independent predictor of coronary disease symptoms. A large Japanese study of over 73,000 men and women showed that feeling stressed is associated with an increased mortality from strokes in women, and with the incidence of coronary disease in both men and women (for the highest stressed women, the stroke risk was more than doubled and the heart disease risk was 60 percent greater than in the lowest stressed women).

High stress affects the susceptibility to cardiac diseases, as well as their progression and ultimate outcome. Various techniques for relaxation to reduce the effects of stress can significantly contribute to prevention and reversal of cardiovascular disorders, including hypertension, strokes, heart attacks, and postsurgery recovery. Valuable techniques include self-hypnosis, meditation, visualization exercises, "relaxation response" practices (as described by Herbert Benson), yoga, and breathing exercises.

A study of thirty-four patients with hypertension showed that yoga relaxation exercise was more effective at reducing blood pressure than less structured relaxation. Blood pressures dropped in the yoga group from 168/100 to 141/84 with just this one intervention. Another study of thirty-four hypertensive subjects showed that stress management and relaxation imagery was successful at lowering both systolic and diastolic blood pressures.

As part of your comprehensive heart-health program, whether for prevention or treatment, include some form of regular stress management. It is good to make an effort to cultivate a relaxed attitude throughout your daily activities, not just at the times when you have a structured meditation or yoga practice. Setting aside twenty minutes of relaxation time daily is valuable for your heart and immune system, but being relaxed at other times is also important.

Exercise and the Heart

Regular exercise is a valuable health practice in many ways; it protects the heart both in prevention and as part of cardiac rehab programs. Aerobic exercise helps the arteries by protecting the endothelium, contributing to maintenance of a normal blood pressure, reducing excess weight, and improving blood flow. Increasing blood flow has an added advantage. As blood passes over the artery lining it creates a physical stress on the endothelial cells and stimulates them to produce potent anti-inflammatory substances, in turn reducing atherosclerosis risks.

Some studies suggest that moderate exercise is not sufficient to lower cardiovascular risks. A large British study showed that brisk walking, bowling, golf, and dancing did not provide much benefit to the heart (although other studies suggest that such activities might provide both this and other benefits). This study showed that jogging, hiking, stair climbing, and swimming (all considered vigorous activity) that averaged 54 calories of energy expenditure per day were associated with a 62 percent reduction in heart mortality.

Aerobic exercise refers to activity that raises heart rate significantly, while at the same time staying within your breathing capacity. A good guideline is to be as vigorous as you can until just before you get short of breath, and keep up the exercise at that level for about thirty minutes or more. In practical terms it means to work up a sweat within thirty minutes without getting out of breath. If you get out of breath, you are working too hard. Simply slow down or stop until your breathing is easier, and then continue at a slower pace.

Anyone can do this level of exercise with virtually no risk, because it does not specify the intensity of exercise, but limits you to your current exercise capacity. If you have a significant heart problem, it will most likely lead to shortness of breath before exercising to the point of putting your heart at risk. If you are unable to work up a sweat in the allotted time, you may have to be gentler with your activity and gradually increase the intensity until you become more fit. This will happen as you persist with your program. You will be able to go faster while having the perception that you are not working any harder. The standard advice is to have an evaluation by your doctor before starting any exercise program.

CONCLUSION

Consider all of your options no matter what your health problems, and make informed decisions about the kind of care that you want. If you can't find a doctor who will work with you using dietary supplements or any other alternative to drugs and surgery, you can contact the American College for Advancement in Medicine (ACAM) at 800-532-3688 or through their website at www.acam.org, to locate a doctor in your area who is open to innovative treatments. I also recommend that you look into chelation therapy for heart disease as part of your comprehensive approach to health care. Most ACAM doctors practice chelation therapy, as well as nutrition and dietary supplement therapy.

Using dietary supplements as part of your comprehensive healthcare program for both treatment and prevention of cardiovascular disease is a positive step in the changing healthcare picture. It gives you more control of your life, and puts you in charge of your health. However, it is only a part of the total prevention and treatment program that you need, and you should be sure to include a healthy diet, exercise, and stress management in your daily life.

The more you know about supplements, the more you can work with your health-care provider to manage your health needs. As more doctors become aware of these treatments and add them to their medical skills you will find it easier to get the medical help you want. An increasing number of people worldwide take dietary supplements, and you would do well to join them. It will help you and your family, and anyone who learns from your example.

SELECTED
REFERENCES

Anderson, R.A., et al., Elevated intakes of supplemental chromium improve glucose and insulin variables in individuals with type 2 diabetes. *Diabetes.* 1997 Nov;46(11): 1786–1791.

Appleby, P.N., et al., Hypertension and blood pressure among meat eaters, fish eaters, vegetarians and vegans in EPIC-Oxford. *Public Health Nutr.* 2002 Oct;5(5):645–654.

Boaz, M., et al., Secondary prevention with antioxidants of cardiovascular disease in endstage renal disease (SPACE): Randomised placebo-controlled trial. *Lancet.* 2000 Oct 7;356(9237):1213–1218.

Castano, G., et al., Comparison of the efficacy and tolerability of policosanol with atorvastatin in elderly patients with type II hypercholesterolaemia. *Drugs Aging.* 2003;20(2): 153–163.

Castano, G., et al., Effects of policosanol and lovastatin in patients with intermittent claudication: A double-blind comparative pilot study. *Angiology.* 2003 Jan;54(1):25–38.

Castano, G., et al., Effects of policosanol and lovastatin on lipid profile and lipid peroxidation in patients with dyslipidemia associated with type 2 diabetes mellitus. *Int J Clin Pharmacol Res.* 2002;22(3–4):89–99.

Chappell, L.T. and M. Janson, EDTA chelation therapy in the treatment of vascular disease. *J Cardiovasc Nurs.* 1996 Apr;10(3):78–86.

Dutta, A. and S.K. Dutta, Vitamin E and its role in the prevention of atherosclerosis and carcinogenesis: A review. *J Am Coll Nutr.* 2003 Aug;22(4):258–268.

Ellis, G.R., et al., Neutrophil superoxide anion-generating capacity, endothelial function and oxidative stress in chronic heart failure: Effects of short- and long-term vitamin C therapy. *J Am Coll Cardiol.* 2000 Nov 1;36(5):1474–1482.

Forlani, S., Combination therapy for prevention of atrial fibrillation after coronary artery bypass surgery: A randomized trial of sotalol and magnesium. *Card Electrophysiol Rev.* 2003 Jun; 7(2): 168–171.

Foster, G.D., et al., A randomized trial of a low-carbohydrate diet for obesity. *N Engl J Med.* 2003 May 22;348(21): 2082–2090.

Hirai, N., et al., Insulin resistance and endothelial dysfunction in smokers: Effects of vitamin C. *Am J Physiol Heart Circ Physiol.* 2000 Sep;279(3):H1172–H1178.

Khaw, K.T., et al., Relation between plasma ascorbic acid and mortality in men and women in EPIC-Norfolk prospective study: A prospective population study. European Prospective Investigation into Cancer and Nutrition. *Lancet.* 2001 Mar 3;357(9257):657–663.

Munkholm, H., et al., Coenzyme Q_{10} treatment in serious heart failure. *Biofactors.* 1999;9(2-4):285–289.

Osganian S.K., et al., Vitamin C and risk of coronary heart disease in women. *J Am Coll Cardiol.* 2003 Jul 16;42(2):246-52.

Pauly, D.F. and C. Pepine, D-Ribose as a supplement for cardiac energy metabolism. *J Cardiovasc Pharmacol Ther.* 2000 Oct;5(4):249–258.

Pereira, M.A., et al., Effect of whole grains on insulin sensitivity in overweight hyperinsulinemic adults. *Am J Clin Nutr.* 2002 May;75(5):848–855.

Rector, T.S., et al., Randomized, double-blind, placebo-controlled study of supplemental oral L-arginine in patients with heart failure. *Circulation.* 1996 Jun 15;93(12):2135–2141.

Ridker, P.M., et al., C-reactive protein and other markers of inflammation in the prediction of cardiovascular disease in women. *N Engl J Med.* 2000 Mar 23;342(12):836–843.

Singh, R.B., et al., A randomised, double-blind, placebo-controlled trial of L-carnitine in suspected acute myocardial infarction. *Postgrad Med J.* 1996 Jan;72(843):45–50.

Singh, R.B., et al., Effect of coenzyme Q_{10} on risk of atherosclerosis in patients with recent myocardial infarction. *Mol Cell Biochem.* 2003 Apr;246(1–2):75–82.

Singh, R.B., et al., Usefulness of antioxidant vitamins in suspected acute myocardial infarction (the Indian experiment of infarct survival-3) *Am J Cardiol.* 1996 Feb 1; 77(4): 232–236.

Steffen, L.M., et al., Associations of whole-grain, refined-grain, and fruit and vegetable consumption with risks of all-cause mortality and incident coronary artery disease and ischemic stroke: The Atherosclerosis Risk in Communities (ARIC) Study. *Am J Clin Nutr.* 2003 Sep;78(3):383–390.

Tice, J.A., et al., Cost-effectiveness of vitamin therapy to lower plasma homocysteine levels for the prevention of coronary heart disease: Effect of grain fortification and beyond. *JAMA.* 2001 Aug 22–29;286(8):936–943.

Wannamethee, S.G. and A.G. Shaper, Taking up regular drinking in middle age: Effect on major coronary heart disease events and mortality. *Heart.* 2002 87: 32–36.

OTHER BOOKS
AND RESOURCES

Botanical Influences on Illness, by Melvin Werbach, M.D. and Michael Murray, N.D. (Third Line Press, Tarzana, California, 1994).

Dr. Janson's New Vitamin Revolution, by Michael Janson, M.D., (Penguin-Putnam/Avery, New York, 2000).

Encyclopedia of Natural Medicine, by Michael Murray, N.D. and Joseph Pizzorno, N.D. (Prima Publishing, Rocklin, California, 1991).

The Inflammation Syndrome, by Jack Challem (Wiley, New York, 2003).

Syndrome X: The Complete Nutritional Program to Prevent and Reverse Insulin Resistance, by J. Challem, B. Berkson, and M.D. Smith (Wiley, New York, 2000).

GreatLife Magazine
Consumer magazine with articles on vitamins, minerals, herbs, and foods.
Available for free at many health and natural food stores.

The Nutrition Reporter™ newsletter
Monthly newsletter that summarizes recent medical research on vitamins, minerals, and herbs.

Customer service:
P.O. Box 30246
Tucson, AZ 85751-0246
e-mail: jack@thenutritionreporter.com
www.nutritionreporter.com

Subscriptions: 12 issues per year, $26 in the U.S.; $32 U.S. or $48 CNC for Canada; $38 for other countries.

Online Resources

Dr. Michael Janson's Website: www.drjanson.com

Updates of the medical literature, editorials, answers to commonly asked questions, and a free monthly newsletter available by email, or submission of individual questions of general interest.

Dr. Michael Janson's Healthy Living

A monthly newsletter on health, nutrition, and integrative medicine. This is a free newsletter posted on Dr. Janson's website, or available by email after signing up at www.drjanson.com.

American College for Advancement in Medicine: www.acam.org

Information about conferences in integrative medicine and a referral source if you are looking for doctors who are familiar with nutrition and vitamins, and practice other forms of integrative medicine, including chelation therapy.

QCI Nutritionals: www.qcinutritionals.com

A mail-order source of high-quality dietary supplements. Also available by phone at 888-922-4848.

Health World Online: www.healthy.net

A comprehensive resource for health information with expert opinions and libraries of information, book excerpts, and articles.

Life Extension Foundation: www.lef.org

A source of articles on health, health politics, and dietary supplements.

National Center for Complementary and Alternative Medicine:
(www.altmed.od.nih.gppov/nccam)
A center of the National Institutes of Health for research and dissemination of information about alternative medicine.

INDEX

Carbohydrates, 15, 72–74
  low intake, 72, 74
Cardiomyopathy, 39, 44
Cerebrovascular
  disease, 66
Chelation therapy for
  circulation, 65–67
Cholesterol, 15, 20, 23,
  26, 47, 49, 54–55, 60
  high-density (HDL),
  15, 20, 23, 27, 34,
  47–48, 50, 53
  low-density (LDL), 20,
  23, 27, 47–48, 50, 67
Cholestin, 49
Chromium, 34–35, 59, 61
  GTF, 35
  picolinate, 35
Cigarette smoke, 15–16,
  30
Citrus bioflavonoids, 59
Cobalamin. *See* Vitamin
  B$_{12}$.
Coenyzme Q$_{10}$, 36–38,
  48, 50, 61–64
Coffee. *See* Caffeine.
Commission E, 53
Copper, 59
C-reactive protein. *See*
  CRP.
Crohn's disease, 24
CRP, 19, 21, 23, 49, 53, 61
Curcumin, 53–54, 62

D'Adamo, Peter J.,
  74–75
Dairy products, 68, 72
Dental disease, 18
Depression, 28
DHA (docosahexaenoic
  acid), 41, 43
Diabetes, 16, 18, 35, 37
Diastole, 4, 9
Diet,1–2, 14–15, 17, 68–77
  fads, 72–75
Digitalis, 44
DNA, 22–25, 50

D-ribose, 50–51, 62–64

Edema, 11
EDTA, 65–67
  oral treatment with,
  66
EFAs, 41–44
Eicosapentaenoic acid
  (EPA), 41, 43
Ejection fraction, 10
EKG, 6, 38
Electrocardiogram. *See*
  EKG.
Endocardium, 4
Endothelial-derived
  relaxing factor, 45
Endothelium, 5, 7, 22,
  29–30, 47, 76
Energy, 39
Enzymes, 32
EPA. *See*
  Eicosapentaenoic
  acid (EPA).
Erectal dysfunction, 46
Essential fatty acids.
  See EFAs.
Estrogen, 19
Ethylene diamine
  tetraacetic acid.
  See EDTA.
Exercise, 1–2, 15, 17, 57,
  76–77
  aerobic, 76–77

Family history and heart
  disease, 13
Fatigue, 29
Fats, 14, 68–70
  polyunsaturated, 70
  saturated, 68
  trans-, 70
Fiber, 73
Fish, 14, 68
  oils, 42–43, 61–64
Flavonoids, 53, 55–56
Flour, white, 14, 69
Fluid accumulation, 11

www.ingramcontent.com/pod-product-compliance
Lightning Source LLC
Jackson TN
JSHW011406130125
77033JS00023B/873